Prekarisierung und soziale Entkopplung – transdisziplinäre Studien

Series Editors

Rolf-Dieter Hepp, Institut für Soziologie, FU Berlin, Berlin, Germany

Robert Riesinger, Journalismus und Public Relations (PR), FH Joanneum Gesellschaft mbH, Graz, Austria

David Kergel, Internationale Hochschule, Duisburg, Germany

Birte Heidkamp-Kergel, E-Learning Zentrum, Hochschule Rhein-Waal, Kamp-Lintfort, Germany

Die Zunahme sozialer Unsicherheit und kultureller Verunsicherung in post-fordistischen Gesellschaften erzeugt einen Status Quo, in dem Prozesse der Prekarisierung und der „sozialen Entkopplung" (Robert Castel) verstärkt das Zentrum der Gesellschaft durchziehen. Der Verlust sozialer Garantien führt dabei zur Aushöhlung sozialstaatlicher Errungenschaften. Dadurch werden die Lebenskontexte und das Alltagsleben der Menschen stark verändert. Das sozialwissenschaftliche Netzwerk S.U.P.I. beschäftigt sich auf europäischer Ebene seit Jahren mit den gegenwärtigen Formen von sozialer Unsicherheit, Prekarität und Ungleichheit. Die Reihe, herausgegeben von Mitgliedern des Netzwerks, präsentiert transdisziplinäre Forschungen zu den sozialen und kulturellen Transformationen in den sozialstaatlich geprägten Demokratien. Sie versteht sich als Forum für die Diskussion in nationalen, europäischen und auch globalen Kontexten. Ebenen einer kritischen Analyse aus multidisziplinären und feldorientierten Perspektiven werden dabei initiiert, aufgenommen und unterstützt. Überschreitung und Öffnung dienen programmatisch als Wegmarken für theoretisch-analytische Beiträge und empirisch-angewandte Forschung.

The increase of social insecurity in post-Fordist societies effect fundamental societal changes. As a consequence Precarity and Disaffiliation (Robert Castel) affecting increasingly the center of society. The loss of social guarantees leads to an erosion of the welfare state. As a result, living situations and everyday life are deeply changed. The S.U.P.I.-Project (Social Uncertainty, Precarity, Inequality) is an European Research Group established by European and international scholars and experts. The network has been concerned with present forms of social insecurity, precariousness and inequality at European level for years. Edited by members of the network, the book series presents transdisciplinary research on aspects of social and cultural transformations in the democracies which are characterized by the welfare state. The book series opens a discursive space for discussions in national, European and global contexts. The contributions of the book series provide critical analyses from multidisciplinaryperspectives, theoretical-analytical reflections and empirical-applied research.

Peter Herrmann

Pandemics as Matter of a System Crisis

Precarity of Society

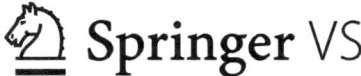 Springer VS

Peter Herrmann
Human Rights Centre
Central South University
Changsha, PR China

ISSN 2509-3266   ISSN 2509-3274 (electronic)
Prekarisierung und soziale Entkopplung – transdisziplinäre Studien
ISBN 978-3-658-43449-6   ISBN 978-3-658-43450-2 (eBook)
https://doi.org/10.1007/978-3-658-43450-2

This Springer VS imprint is published by the registered company Springer Fachmedien Wiesbaden
GmbH, part of Springer Nature.
The registered company address is: Abraham-Lincoln-Str. 46, 65189 Wiesbaden, Germany

Paper in this product is recyclable.

We are often compelled to set up standards we cannot reach ourselves, and to lay down rules which we could not ourselves satisfy. … It is not needful to point out the awful danger of admitting the principle which has been contended for. Who is to be the judge of this sort of necessity?

(Lord Coleridge, judge in Queen v Dudley and Stephens)

I am grateful for comments but also for debates and encouragement throughout the recent month, directly and indirectly inspiring – and sometimes this means – provoking thoughts that are reflected in the elaboration.
The members of the working group HRUG, namely 黎娟, 郭敏, 毛俊响, 盛喜, George Mpedi Lethlokwa, Joseph Finnerty, Mehmet Okyayuz, Nuria Pumar Beltran and Arno Tausch.
Invaluable comments and inspirations I owe to Beate Hoffmann and Jacob Kornbeck.
Not least I am thanking Rolf Hepp, editor of the series and Cori Antonia Mackrodt from Springer-publishing house for their openness to accept the somewhat unconventional work, and still helping with some constructive comments on a first submission.

Foreword

Political Scientist, Department of Political Science and Public Administration, Faculty of Economic and Administrative Sciences, Middle East Technical University, Ankara/Turkey

The present text by Peter Herrmann locates the pandemic crisis, which began in March 2020 and has still not come to an end despite all the attempts to overcome it, in a wide-ranging framework of biological, medical and above all social and political contexts. Herrmann puts it this way: 'While biological, medical, differentiated social impact-assessments are delivering at most some background melodies, these issues are here back-staged, behind the main scene of the—in the widest sense—political topic; however, this political field is itself taken in a wide approach, implying historical, power- and democracy-theoretical questions and the like.'

The fact that the peak of the main period of the pandemic occurred from late 2020 to early 2021 meant that political aspects were all too quickly forgotten over time. Since then, from the author's point of view, it became necessary to speak not only of a purely medical virus but also of a political virus that makes people sick not only from a medical perspective, but from a citizen's perspective. Herrmann states: '...opening the eyes to see that another virus, not less dangerous than the Corona-virus, is already for a long time in place, and made the German polity to what it is today: a precarious political system, an illness that makes many citizens sick'. This connection is an expression of a systemic crisis, which will be dealt with in detail in the further course of the text, in particular from a legal and institutional point of view. This is part of the mentioned classification into an overall political and soci(et)al context, which transfers the author's pedagogical-subjective concerns, as showing his foreign students specific mechanisms for dealing with a pandemic within the political and legal framework in the

Federal Republic of Germany, from a purely individualistic to a structural level. A particular approach aimed at medical solutions is thus contextualised and elevated to a holistic level. Above all, it is also about showing that the pandemic represents an extreme situation, but that the political virus is always carried along in the everyday structures of German politics and thus also represents a permanent, albeit 'dormant', disease of the Federal Republican system and its citizens. An approach that is to be welcomed, all the more so when one considers how much the fight against the pandemic in the public (or better: published) debate has all too often been presented as a purely technical-administrative package of measures. Such presentation is itself an expression of this polity, which has been degraded to a 'management system' for a long time or was perhaps even aspired to by the Allies after the Second World War. Only in the recent past—albeit mostly with the omission of democratic-theoretical and thus also of human rights concerns—has the bringing together of the most diverse aspects been made a little more of an issue. However, the merit of the present text is that it brings the different perspectives in a way together that is less concerned with soliciting cheap applause from the (critical) public; instead it provides a theoretical and social scientifically sound analysis of the pandemic crisis. When reading the text, the almost forgotten tradition of a critical social science came to my mind, which does not understand the essence of reality as a mere listing of individual facts, but rather aims to classify them in the already mentioned—also historical—overall context. Already this reminder deserves appreciation.

Understanding this overall context also requires (re)thinking the complexity of the relationship between the individual and society, and its various forms of interaction and mediation within and across various levels, including the institutional one. A modern example of such thinking is the much-quoted statement by Marx that the individual does not exist as an independent unit, but only in the ensemble of social conditions. Herrmann brings this thesis 'up to date' by making reference to Leo Kofler's subject-object conceptualization. This approach generally runs throughout the text, aiming at avoiding an individualized and often abstract approach to the subject. In this context—I think—the often long original quotations in the text must also be understood: The author is also guided by a didactic concern. And the recourse to reading 'between the lines' is brought to mind again and again with very long quotes.

The human rights issues inherent in the pandemic crisis have manifested themselves from the start, particularly in the context of socio-economic inequality. In the last three years, the precarization of ever broader social classes has progressed further and further. Parallel to this development, which is still based in principle on the contradiction between capital and labour, tendencies can and could be ascertained which attempt to present this development as detached, quasi-independent of bourgeois-capitalist structures. At this point the author reminds the reader again, another time showing connections within the overall context, that structural aspects of social reality appear modified in their details, but are still generally valid. In this context, the author uses the pandemic crisis, which is very present in social consciousness, as the initial spark for such a recontextualization—critical analysis meets once again a didactical plan.

This intention is realized by conceptualizing the problem of alienation, supplemented by the aspect of institutional and political alienation, whose 'overall effect is an increasing societal efficiency, going hand in hand with a decreasing societal meaning'.

Drug research is perhaps the most concrete expression of this far-reaching topic of alienation in the context of global political power constellations. Questions of production and reproduction, but also of jurisdiction and their social and political responsibility collide here. For Herrmann, this development culminates in the fact that drug discovery has become part of a geopolitical strategy, with health reduced to a management issue.

The universality of the human rights question is conveyed only in a very abbreviated and thus insufficient manner via a process of 'technicalization': '... from technicalization of the problematique by which inequalities (being affected by the disease, consequences of the disease, access to treatment, supply shortages . ..) are reduced on technical issues that can easily be solved and do not need political solutions. It is the subsequent 'perpetuation of slavery' that is as such a breach of human rights. And, indeed, from here we can also make out a breach of human rights as a matter of suppression of freedom of speech. But far from being mainly a matter of limiting public gatherings etc., the technicalization is part of a structural shortcoming of today's socio-economic constellation of polities: the lack of (space for) discourse.' Here Herrmann closes the arc that he draws across the entire text within the framework of the relationship between the individual and society, from the right to individual concerns to the need to strive for 'a culture of open dispute'.

I understand Herrmann's remarks as a kind of basic text, which should make it possible to conceptually grasp the events in the current pandemic period in their soci(et)al totality. The freedom of the individual in relation to a collective responsibility for the common good of society is dealt with in the further course of the text using the examples of the Chinese constitution and the social responsibility requirement of property in the Basic Law of Germany. This is followed by comments on the Irish, Turkish and South African constitutions regarding this mostly fraught relationship.

One line of the 'structural dimension of the Corona Crisis' that runs through the text is its linkage to human rights issues. In this context, four strands are dealt with: Power, Knowledge, Caring for Life and Escape into Living. We can call the above-mentioned techniques of analysis a multi-layered approach.

As a kind of summary of this approach, the following words by Herrmann must be highlighted: 'In short, the Corona crisis turns out to be a disclosure of the precarity of the current socio-political system, confronting societal actors on all levels with the questioning of the hitherto accepted system, the fundamental consensus—this time not by ideologies or different groups asking for the change of realities but by changed realities demanding a new understanding thereof. Such different understanding is, however, not a matter of theory but an understanding of what must be done by whom and for whom. As such it is ultimately both, relational and self-enhancing. We find these processes on all three levels, i.e. the micro-, meso- and macro-level, thus resulting in a new analytical approach to precarity: it is the helplessness, or better: the inappropriateness of a socio-institutional system that lost its legitimation as consequence of the ultimate bond to use-value.'

This also makes clear that this work represents an important contribution to the discussion about precarity and precarization; in a nutshell: Precarization certainly affects individuals or certain 'social groups'. However, precariousness is a basic disease of the socio-political and political-economic system, the roots of which can be located long before and much deeper than today's mostly labour market-related discussion often suggests.

Beyond all that has been mentioned, key points of philosophical-theoretical as well as sociological thinking can be found throughout the text. The organization of society should, of course, also include the legal component, since otherwise it remains trapped in its 'own reflection' or runs the risk of being reduced to 'contractual relationships between—natural or legal—personalities'. By pointing out that this necessary sociality of law is too often omitted, Herrmann paints a dystopia of the rule of law in its mainstream interpretation 'as state of the fittest'. The resulting 'competitive society' is not prevented or mitigated when politicians like Angela Merkel publicize the will to be able to do as narrative. But at least this narrative in the context of migration policy was—at least in part—motivating enough to initiate social organization by the members of society themselves. This was made even easier by the fact that the institutional framework for the implementation of this social organization was in place. Exactly this component, which institutionally (and also constitutionally) supports social responsibility and personal initiative, was missing during the pandemic crisis. Herrmann makes this clear by the pointing out the insufficient involvement of the legislature in decision-making processes to combat the pandemic. This circumvention was practiced on the basis of mechanisms such as the Infection Protection Act, which, according to Herrmann, actually represents a kind of emergency legislation. Shutdowns and the limitation of social activities were some of the measures. The overall context in which all this has to be classified is wide-ranging and corresponds to the current global situation of inequality at the national level. However, Herrmann differs from other critical voices in that he does not fundamentally reject the need for 'restrictions'; In addition to the references to the lack of legitimacy through procedures, he emphasizes that it must ultimately be about a fundamentally different orientation: the freedom of society is more and different than an aggregate of the freedom and licentiousness of individuals.

Herrmann: 'The general notion of living in a performance and competition society had now been complemented by the notion of a society of distrust. After the questionable promise of 'blossoming landscapes' as result of the so-called unification, the pandemic confronted the population another time with promises turning out as questionable: the assurance of socio-physical security, guaranteed by a well-developed and expensive social insurance and the reality of a health threat for which nobody would sign responsible, on the contrary: governments and businesses feeling themselves uncomfortably threatened, while the quest for responsible actors increased. An attitude of fear, panic, egoism and egocentrism continued in one way or another—the mindset itself did not change, only the framework changed, leading to even more pronounced expressions. The fact of the structural character of failures and contradictions became obvious in various ways—not least by the opposition equally lacking constructivist proposals.'

Herrmann points out that the legitimacy of state actions is in this way reduced on a technical-procedural dimension. It is therefore no longer constantly discussed anew through social discourse, perhaps even ideally constantly newly created, but 'determined' by state authorities. In this way, the socio-economic consequences of fighting the pandemic are also covered up and reduced to a dimension that can no longer be questioned. Short-time work and the problem of online work, to name just two examples, with all the negative consequences for social groups that are already disadvantaged, are widening the gap between rich and poor. The principles of the welfare state collide with this, but are only launched as secondary in view of the priorities to combat the pandemic, which enjoy the highest existential esteem.

At this point, Herrmann also looks at the role of the media and their function as necessary initiators and companions of a public critical discourse. This discourse, already presented in classical texts such Habermas' analysis of the bourgeois public sphere as a prerequisite for an enlightened and enlightened modernity, has come to an end, or—to put it more moderately—has been marginalized.

With its intertwining of different perspectives, including personal experience, Herrmann's text is suitable for raising the memory of what seems to have been forgotten—it is a contribution to the culture of remembrance. He makes clear the upheavals during the ongoing pandemic crisis, which are increasingly making up the structure of civil society without being able to properly recognize and locate their importance. It is no exaggeration to say that his text pretends to disavow the attempt—perhaps unprecedented in its form—at an ideological redefinition and consolidation of existing unequal relationships. All credit is due to such an attempt, and I wish the text many readers.

Mehmet Okyayuz

Aversion to Affection

Often books had been introduced by a dedication or affection to the reader—an expression of the authors' recognition of the subject of work, the appreciation of the reader and respect towards the author himself. While all this is also guiding the presentation of the current work, it may need some qualification: • regarding the recognition of the subject, the Corona virus, it is admitted, that this work can only reflect a tiny part of the entire subject matter and is, at the same time, going beyond a narrow interpretation. While biological, medical, differentiated social impact-assessments are delivering at most some background melodies, these issues are here back-staged, behind the main scene of the—in the widest sense—political topic; however, this political field is itself taken in a wide approach, implying historical, power- and democracy-theoretical questions and the like; • regarding the appreciation of the reader, it is surely guiding underlying the analysis and presentation, but it means not least to challenge the reader, asking for the readiness to follow the walk on some hidden trails and somewhat long and winded roads; • finally, looking at the author's self-respect, it is not afflicted in principal terms; however, it is respectfully confined by the knowledge of the limits of possible knowledge and the impossibility to resolve all contradictions of life and living. Against this backdrop the following must be understood also as dedication to foreign students at the Berlin School of Economics and Law, to whom I gave lectures about *History, Politics and Economics of the Host Country:* it had been about rejecting the computer wisdom of the windows generation: *WYSI-WYG—What you see is what you get.* Real life had been, is and will be not least shaped by the hidden small print in conjunction with the big lines of polities—the rest is metaphor, application along the motto of *The Leopard*, who left Sicily a long time ago, preaching that *Se vogliamo che tutto rimanga come è, bisogna che tutto cambi.—Everything must change for everything to remain the same' (Giuseppe Tomasi di Lampedusa: Il Gattopardo)*— the motto of polity changes today.

Contents

Pandemics as Matter of a System Crisis—Precarity of Society

While Corona is still the topic also in the perspective of virology and medicine, it seems to be justified to say that the urgency of pandemic's is not anymore given to the extent as it had been the case at the end of 2020/the beginning of 2021. On the political agenda, while it is not completely virus-free, the topic crossed as well its peak. While all this must be taken with caution, it seems at this stage more important to look at some fundamental issues, emerging on different levels and in different circles—the reader will hopefully follow the author on the way to look behind the curtain of the pandemics, opening the eyes to see that another virus, not less dangerous than the Corona-virus, is already for a long time in place, and made the German polity to what it is today: a precarious political system, an illness that makes many citizens sick.

It is especially clear that issues of societal formation, the political institutional system and not least the question of human rights came to the fore. In particular the issue of human rights emerged in more concrete forms, elevated considerations about abstract principles in a new frame and against a new background: Instead of looking at general matters of individuality, freedom, democracy etc.. these topics emerged as concerns of every day's life within global governance, national polities, social strata and families; behind the veil of objective criteria and expertise, personal relationships and institutional settings faced destructive verification.

The present book aims on understanding political processes in this tensional perspective, on the one hand being seemingly matters of daily decisions in parliamentary processes, being on the other hand issues of most fundamental questions

P. Herrmann, *Pandemics as Matter of a System Crisis,* Prekarisierung und soziale Entkopplung – transdisziplinäre Studien, https://doi.org/10.1007/978-3-658-43450-2_1

of human rights, and even the understanding of the essence of rights. The problematique of this discussion is given by the fact that rights can only be understood if they are related to obligations, and as such elementary forms of society and social relationships. In other words, we are dealing with a complex field of individual behaviour, interrelationality and institutional framing—all being a matter of processuality.

Part of this is another dialectic, namely that of subject and object. In a very pronounced way, Leo Kofler makes us aware of this by highlighting the process of intermediation and its meaning for the subject t-object-relationship. In his words:

> The theory of the subject-object relationship can be summarised as follows: In his actions, the human individual (the subject) 'produces' actions and relationships directed towards the achievement of concrete goals, which in their totality condense into an ordered system (object), which in turn confronts the human being as a system of conditions (subject) and determines him in his actions (whereby the human being in turn becomes an object). The objective character of 'environment', which is 'produced' by man himself, thus becomes subjective in turn by degrading man to an object, but at the same time setting him new tasks and stimulating him to new activity that changes the circumstances, to activity as a subject. The concrete content of this relationship (identity of the subjective and the objective) depends on the concrete character of social development itself.
>
> (Kofler: 44 f.; own translation)

Decisive is that this 'legal' subject-object relationship of a particular epoch includes all phenomena, starting with the simplest economic facts up to the most complicated intellectual creations and is in this way the core of 'man making his own history'.

The often-cited principles of human rights, namely universality, inalienability, indivisibility, interdependence and interrelatedness, are gaining in this light a new relevance: without feeding into historical (or social) relativism, we arrive at valuable statements only by acknowledging the ecologies of scale, scope and action of law, not least meaning the consideration of justice as use value, standing behind the juridical expressions of law which occurs as exchange value. In other words, we refer to the patterns of scale (a), of scope (b) and action (c), well known from economics. It is proposed to apply this to jurisprudence, in this case a specific ecology of norms, referring to the study of the household in its relation to the surrounding and the relational management (use of resources ....)—with this we have a very close link to the economy, also originating in the approach to managing the household. As such, it is not about simple sets of rules; instead, we are looking at power constellations, where power is defined by and caught in the tensional field of appropriateness in the dialectical twofold function of reflecting and relating to the given conditions and subsequently their subordination.

Thus, we are talking about responsibility as well as the availability of spaces for which we are responsible, making and maintaining them as spaces where life can be lived.

Against this background it should be clear that the topic is closely linked to precarity—not only and not even primarily because people working in precarious positions and those facing precarious living conditions have more problems than people living in stable conditions. While eating strawberries throughout the year sounds tempting, such availability is only one marked—and marketed—example of a general development closely linked to and underlying, though as such often overlooked matter, processes of precarisation: • in economic terms the quasi-separation of use and exchange value, • with this the thorough establishment of wage labour and the subsequent truncation of labour process from the worker in the sense of the more or less complete commodification of the labour force, • and thus the alienation as principle determining societal processes, with • finally defining political processes as quasi-independent from real societal processes, following reflexive rules that guarantee reproduction, • thus drawing the circle of what is reproduced increasingly tight, comparable with economic processes which arrived with the recent financialisation a new stage of detachment of what the economy is actually about, namely the production and reproduction of people's and peoples' daily life. Precarisation is, then, understood as four-level process of hyper-alienation:

(A) Labour Alienation
   • alienation of the worker from use-value led processes of production
   • truncation of exchange-value led activities from use-value led productions
(B) Economic Alienation
   • alienation of the exchange-value led productive processes from use value production
   • truncation of managing from regulating and controlling productive processes
(C) Organisational Alienation
   • alienation of organisations from set goals and objectives as result of 'administrative sovereignty'
   • truncation of management tasks and their externalisation
(D) Political Alienation
   • alienation of management from requirements of regulation of life and living

- truncation of a self-reflexive political system, oriented towards and defined by the goal of maintenance of power, establishing itself as politico-administrative system, increasingly independent from the socio-economic fabrique.

The overall effect is an increasing societal efficiency, going hand in hand with a decreasing societal meaning—or more in technical terms: feedback loops are oriented along the lines of internal functioning of a closely knit and bordered system, with subsequent precarity as long and to the extent to which the claimed and supposed goals cannot be realised.

Preparing the Ground for an Economic Perspective

2

The problematique became particularly clear with the beginning of the pandemics, especially at the stage of the manifestation of the harsh consequences of the virus in connection with the need to redefine both, statutory responsibilities (and even the need of revisiting the questions of who and what falls under 'statutory bodies') and the scope of their responsibility and power to act and/or even coordinate action. Moreover, even the question of how responsibility can be localised in the tensional field between individual development and self-fulfilment on the one hand and soci(et)al obligation and commitment towards the common weal on the other hand had to be moved to the fore. It must be said, though, that speaking of such tension is misleading if taken as eternal matter. Here, and in general, when looking at (human) rights, it is important to consider what Karl Marx stated in the first volume of Capital, arguing against Proudhon, namely that he

> *begins by taking his ideal of Justice, of 'justice éternelle', from the juridical relations that correspond to the production of commodities: thereby, it may be noted, he proves, to the consolation of all good citizens, that the production of commodities is a form of production as everlasting as justice. Then he turns round and seeks to reform the actual production of commodities, and the actual legal system corresponding thereto, in accordance with this ideal. ... Do we really know any more about 'usury', when we say it contradicts 'justice éternelle', 'équité éternelle', 'mutualité éternelle', and other 'vérités éternelles' than the fathers of the church did when they said it was incompatible with 'grâce éternelle', 'foi éternelle', and 'la volonté éternelle de Dieu'?*

(Marx, 1867: 96)

P. Herrmann, *Pandemics as Matter of a System Crisis,* Prekarisierung und soziale Entkopplung – transdisziplinäre Studien, https://doi.org/10.1007/978-3-658-43450-2_2

Marx' critique is—taking a juridical perspective—not least directed against the understanding of rights as formalism, following a binary code: the supposed ideal world of the 'eternal good', positioned against the supposed evil, in Christianity incarnated by the devil, incarcerating his victims in the purgatory of an inescapable oppression, in the spirit of capitalism encoded as capital, of which Katharina Pistor says that it

> is coded in law. Ordinary assets are just that—a plot of land, a promise to be paid in the future, the pooled resources from friends and family to set up a new business, or individual skills and know-how. Yet every one of these assets can be transformed into capital by cloaking it in the legal modules that were also used to code asset-backed securities and their derivatives, which were at the core of the rise of finance in recent decades. These legal modules, namely contract, property rights, collateral, trust, corporate, and bankruptcy law, can be used to give the holders of some assets a comparative advantage over others.
>
> (Pistor, 2019: X)

Thus

> [h]ere is how capitalism actually works — use a legal framework of private ownership to extract value from the labor of others. The end game is a system that hoards wealth, stifles innovation, and ultimately destroys the value created by cooperation among those who seek to do things that cannot be done alone.
>
> (Brever, 2016)

Taking issues like legality/justice, particularism/universalism etc. into account, it is useful to enter the debate on property. By looking at small property holders, we get easily distracted from the real question, namely the meaning of property in respect of production—we must remember that production is understood as (re-)production of daily life of people. This is of special importance when it comes to human rights, as it is here, where decisions are taken: decisions not only concerning the proprietor and the deployment of workforce, but also other people, society at large, and the environment—all understood by taking relationality and processuality into account. This gains even new dimensions with production in general and capitalist process of valorisation in particular gain new dimensions: after a—relative—demeaning of the primary, the secondary and the tertiary sector we reached a stage where 'Efficiently manufacturing things that people wanted was no longer enough. People's desires were themselves a product requiring skillful manufacture.' (Varoufakis, Feb 23, 2022) This de-materialisation of the material process of the economy means not least that law—and behind it obscene power—gains the ultimate meaning and control: While at least a piece of mud stands behind the processes referred to by Pistor, we are now talking about air or even less. Still, it is 'expensive' or better said: made expensive. This is true not only in monetary terms but also in terms of human lives as could be seen in the performance of the pharmaceutical industry.

> *Bayer is a good example. The company had shelved basic pharmaceutical research long before the 'high priority' strategy announced in the mid-2000s. And it was by no means only anti-infectives that fell victim to the turnaround carried out with its implementation. The pill producer also gave up the search for new antibiotics, despite the increasingly frequent resistance of pathogens to the old drugs. Preparations that people are only allowed to take for a certain period of time simply do not pay off. 'We have to earn money with our products. This means that not all the medicines we need are developed', with these words former CEO Marijn Dekkers once outlined the political economy of the medicine business in a Spiegel interview in 2015. In order to comply with this, the global player develops lots of pharmaceuticals that nobody needs instead of urgently needed medicines. It even manages to invent diseases such as the 'menopause of men' when new sales markets need to be created.*

> *(Perke, 2021: 296 f.; with reference to: Pauly/Dohmen, 2015).*

Against this backdrop, research in medication against the virus had been taken up late, then, however, under high pressure—at the end using the results in a geopolitical strategy of which the winner had been known at the outset: the major players of the pharmaceutical sector. It does not come as a surprise to see articles in the predominantly conservative mass media, namely the German FAZ, considering socialisation as legitimate means, enforcing socially responsible use of the means of production. If outspoken or not, this reflects the fact that problems are in fact depoliticised: as long as capitalism is fighting for its existence, it is confronted with matters that it cannot solve, moreover that are inherently emerging from its own contradictions. The solution proposed by the very same system is the elaboration of a technical approach, based on a technical definition of health, inequality, government, living together, support etc.. Such managerial approach to the social is, however, misleading as it is not questioning the structural issues causing the dysfunctions, or we may say 'the a-social of the social'. Making the slave voice-less enforces the perpetuation of the master–slave relationship in the Hegelian understanding:

> *Yet, the Master is not quite the master and the Slave is not quite the slave. The Master wants to be freely recognized as Master. But the Slave only acknowledges him as such because he is enslaved. Recognition is not freely given. The Master controls the Slave. But the Slave, in making himself the physical form of the Master's will, in turn*

exercises control over the Master. It is his work that makes the Master's life possible. The Master is increasingly alienated from the world that the Slave creates for him, precisely because it is a world created by another. The Slave, on the other hand, begins to see himself reflected in the world he is creating and, unlike the Master, finds recognition through his labour. The Master, having become wholly dependent upon the world created by the Slave, finds himself enslaved by that world. The Slave is still a slave, with no freedom. The Master is the master, with total freedom. And, yet, their relationship has subtly and profoundly changed, as have the meanings of freedom and enslavement.

(Malik, 2014)

In this light, the breaches of Human Rights, often mentioned in the context of Corona politics, should primarily not be seen as matter of suppression of opinions and the like. Instead, breaches emerge from technicalisation of the problematique by which inequalities (being affected by the disease, consequences of the disease, access to treatment, supply shortages …) are reduced on technical issues that can easily be solved and do not need political solutions. It is the subsequent 'perpetuation of slavery' that is as such a breach of Human rights. And, indeed, from here we can also make out a breach of Human Rights as matter of suppression of freedom of speech. But far from being mainly a matter of limiting public gatherings etc., the technicalisation is part of a structural shortcoming of today's socio-economic constellation of polities: the lack of (space for) discourse. This is, however, not as new as we may think at first glance. Gotthold Ephraim Lessing stated in 1769

Not that I don't think our present public is a little too disgusted with everything that is called a polemic and looks like it. They seem to want to forget that the enlightenment of many important points results from mere contradiction, and that people would still not be in agreement about anything in the world if they had not quarrelled about anything in the world.

'Quarrelled'; for that is what kindness calls all quarrelling: and quarrelling has become something so unmannerly that one may be far less ashamed to hate and slander than to quarrel.

If, however, the greater part of the public, which does not want to know of any polemical writings, were writers themselves, it would probably not be the mere politesse that does not want to tolerate the polemical tone. It is so uncomfortable for self-love and self-conceit! It is so dangerous to the fake names! It is so dangerous to the names that have been faked.

But truth, they say, so rarely wins in the process.

(Lessing, 1769: 183; translated P.H.)

In other words, we have to address urgently the general problem of the lack of a culture of open dispute, on the one hand not confrontational, on the other hand not denying and, in any case, transcending individual concern(s).

Approaching an Understanding of Society: Property—Ownership

Looking at relevant definitions in different constitutions is interesting. Articles 12 and 13 of the Chinese Constitution state the following:

Article 12

Socialist public property is inviolable.

The State protects socialist public property. Appropriation or damaging of State or collective property by any organization or individual by whatever means is prohibited.

Article 13

Citizens' lawful private property is inviolable.

The State, in accordance with law, protects the rights of citizens to private property and to its inheritance.

The State may, in the public interest and in accordance with law, expropriate or requisition private property for its use and make compensation for the private property expropriated or requisitioned.

However, more interesting are the preceding articles, beginning with article 6, which sets the framework:

The basis of the socialist economic system of the People's Republic of China is socialist public ownership of the means of production, namely, ownership by the whole people and collective ownership by the working people. The system of socialist public ownership supersedes the system of exploitation of man by man; it applies the principle of 'from each according to his ability, to each according to his work'.

P. Herrmann, *Pandemics as Matter of a System Crisis*, Prekarisierung und soziale Entkopplung – transdisziplinäre Studien, https://doi.org/10.1007/978-3-658-43450-2_3

Finally we read in article 53 that the citizens'

> *must abide by the Constitution and other laws, keep State secrets, protect public property, observe labour discipline and public order and respect social ethics.*

The entire article is presented to show the context in which the reference to property stands.

Then, the German basic law speaks of the social obligation following from property and refers interestingly to both, expropriation and nationalisation. Article 14 reads

[Property—Inheritance—Expropriation]

(1) Property and the right of inheritance shall be guaranteed. Their content and limits shall be defined by the laws.

(2) Property entails obligations. Its use shall also serve the public good.

(3) Expropriation shall only be permissible for the public good. It may only be ordered by or pursuant to a law that determines the nature and extent of compensation. Such compensation shall be determined by establishing an equitable balance between the public interest and the interests of those affected. In case of dispute concerning the amount of compensation, recourse may be had to the ordinary courts.

and article 15 rules

[Nationalisation]

Land, natural resources and means of production may, for the purpose of nationalisation, be transferred to public ownership or other forms of public enterprise by a law that determines the nature and extent of compensation. With respect to such compensation the third and fourth sentences of paragraph (3) of Article 14 shall apply, mutatis mutandis.

The Irish Constitution states in article 43

Private Property

1 1° The State acknowledges that man, in virtue of his rational being, has the natural right, antecedent to positive law, to the private ownership of external goods.

2° The State accordingly guarantees to pass no law attempting to abolish the right of private ownership or the general right to transfer, bequeath, and inherit property.

2 1° The State recognises, however, that the exercise of the rights mentioned in the foregoing provisions of this Article ought, in civil society, to be regulated by the principles of social justice.

2° The State, accordingly, may as occasion requires delimit by law the exercise of the said rights with a view to reconciling their exercise with the exigencies of the common good.

Together with China, the Constitution of South Africa is especially interesting— all the references cannot be presented here. Chapter two, with the headline *Bill of Rights,* has a long article (25), outlining in detail issues that are linked to property (rights). The general provision says

(1) No one may be deprived of property except in terms of law of general application,

and no law may permit arbitrary deprivation of property.

(2) Property may be expropriated only in terms of law of general application—

(a) for a public purpose or in the public interest; and

(b) subject to compensation, the amount of which and the time and manner of payment of which have either been agreed to by those affected or decided or approved by a court.

Sentence (3) to (9) outline the details especially of the conditions of expropriation. Of special interest are sentence (6) and (7) as they refer to property of 'a person or community'.

Other regulations of the constitution are ruling taxation issues, municipal services etc.

Looking at the Turkish constitution we find in article 35 the sentence that.

[e]veryone has the right to own and inherit property. These rights may be limited by law only in view of public interest. The exercise of the right to property shall not contravene public interest.

Of special interest are I this case other references to property rights, namely articles 21 and 23, referring not least to moral obligations and the prevention of crime.

Looking at these different constitutional provisions, we can distinguish at least three patterns: first, and we may say this is a kind of original state, the point of departure is common property—this is as well prioritised, and only subsequently private property is introduced, separated from the commons, while the latter remains prioritised. The other extreme is the prioritisation of private property, only ex post the common wheal is introduced and—depending on the way of its socialisation (expropriation or nationalisation)—we find the specific reasons as well the relevant forms of compensation. Of special interest is that community forms of property and private property are going hand in hand, however, community property remaining apparently a crucial point of reference.

In any case, there is little reference in the constitutions referring to the purpose of property, although the Chinese constitution is in some way an exception, as it defines in broad terms the economy as point of reference. Thinking about a broad enough concept, relevant for further debates on human rights, the following is proposed for further consideration. On the one hand, we find a lose connection to the understanding of John Locke, who emphasised the natural right to property, going hand in hand with it the emphasis that a limit is set by the need of the proprietor and his/her ability to handle it. However, we depart from Locke, as appropriation is in his understanding limited (i) on private production (ii) for private use. For a Human Rights approach this should be revisited: production—in the strict economic sense and as matter of production and reproduction of soci(et)al life—is today to such an extent socialised, that private production is nearly a hoax. The same is true for reproduction, as today reproduction is not only social by way of immediate interaction, but also by a whole set of means, going much beyond immediate interaction and reaching across the globe—in both cases it also depends on means provided by society. It is sufficient to mention only one set of examples, namely the education in schools, the use of social instruments like books, computers, the Internet; increasingly the Internet is becoming itself a means and source of socialisation, coming together with others, depending on artificial intelligence, which emerges itself from social (inter)action and turning more and more into a subject sui generis.[1]

Interesting aspects had been discussed in the early 1950s by German public and constitutional law. Helmut K. J. Ridder, in a prominent presentation during the annual conference of the public policy and international law academics, engaged in the topic expropriation and socialisation, aiming on specifying the terms.[2] Although his contribution had been very much employed by discussing specific issues of the German basic law and it it's articles 14 and 15, it is of general interest. Summarising the highly differentiated analysis, there are two fundamentally different forms: the one aims on specifying the use of property, without actually changing the legal title whereas the other changes the property

---

[1] See for this context Freeman, 2019: 6

[2] Ridder, 1951

title. However, this is only part of the difference. Another, and more important, aspect becomes clear when we follow Ridder's reflection on the motives. The following quote marks the fundamental difference:

> *In the case of expropriation, the de-privatisation of property is also seen on the part of the expropriating state or the state granting the right of expropriation, as it were, with an expression of regret for the affected party, necessary for the sake of the administrative project, because a free contractual settlement was or would be rejected by the affected party or would be practically impossible to implement for other reasons.*

> *In the case of social devaluation, the de-privatisation of the assets of the person effected is decisive, because the private character of the assets is thought to be currently or potentially harmful to society. Compared to this negative purpose of social devaluation, the positive aspects of a general nature (new impulses for the national economy, raising the standard of living of broad strata, etc.) are at most of secondary importance and those of a special nature (increasing the profitability in a certain branch of the economy, etc.) are almost insignificant ... .*

> *(Ridder: 140)*

In short, we see in the one case a measure, that intervenes in each individual case, thus making a specific 'project' possible; in the other case we are witnessing a kind of system-change, independent of an individual case, aiming on a change of a structural issue. It may be in one case, the intervention allowing to build a road, in the other case it would an intervention that allows to structurally influence the availability of accommodation. Another aspect is occasionally added, also in some way proposed by Ridder: the latter case is distinct from nationalisation, transferring ownership—responsibility for care and use—directly to citizens.

Finally, he suggests that subsequently the social devaluation—unlike expropriation is not a legal institution but a legal form, as such part of a fundamental change:

> *Cases, regulated by expropriation, can recur randomly. The state uses expropriation ad hoc. That is why its focus is also ... on the individual act.*

> *The social devaluation has a unique aim; it fulfils the mission of socialisation. The Basic Law expressly permits, as is appropriate to the matter, only the legislative path for social devaluation according to Article 15. And it must be demanded that these laws are reduced on some of the enterprises of a given industrial branch.*

> *(ibid.: 142)*

As much as all this is crucially a matter of the economy, it is important to note, that the establishment of a mindset is going hand in hand with the approaches.

We can easily see that for instance health related behaviour, health services and related issues are influenced by this mindset: the question would then be, if health is considered as something that is secured by society—as citizens' right—or if health must be secured by individuals themselves, being a private matter; the question is on the latter case also, if the individual has in case of transmittable diseases main responsibility towards others. In the given case the backdrop, against which such debate emerges, is clearly given by a strategy document that had been elaborated on behalf of what is now the Federal Ministry of the Interior and Community, then headed by minister Horst Seehofer (https://www.abgeordnetenwatch.de/recherchen/informationsfreiheit/das-int erne-strategiepapier-des-innenministeriums-zur-corona-pandemie; 02/03/2023)— the document had been declared as *'Confidential—For Official Use Only'*. While the severe threat is in no way denied in the document, a worst-case scenario with death toll of 1 million people is presented and it is even stated that concealment is not an option, the principal worry seems to be something else:

> *The German economy is a high-performance machine that year after year provides a high level of material prosperity and public goods accessible to all citizens, such as comprehensive health care and public safety. Its performance is supported by a high degree of division of labour within and outside the country. The prerequisite for this is that the majority of all existing enterprises and workers are operational and that the integrity of the overall system is not called into question.*

> *This is precisely what makes the national economy as vulnerable as a high-performance engine, because only the simultaneous functioning of all its components preserves the viability of the entire system. It is true that in normal operation moderate cyclical fluctuations can be effectively smoothed over time, above all through social security systems. So, as long as the machine is running more or less at full speed, minor disruptions to the system are not a serious problem. Every working day more or less then translates into a slightly larger or smaller GDP in the final accounts. But this 'normal world' is now suspended, we are on uncharted territory.*

> *If the measures proposed here to contain and control the Covid 19 epidemic do not work, the entire system could be called into question in the sense of a 'meltdown'. This threatens to change the community into a completely different ground state, up to and including anarchy.*

> *(ibid.: 8)*

To conclude, we may say that the definition of appropriation must be linked to an elaborated understanding of appropriateness. Politically this can only be realised by developing a multilateral and global approach towards democracy, on the one hand referring to the fact that we are dealing with the global economy, on the other hand equally accepting the diversity when it comes to the mode of production.

This serves well as background and framework for thoroughly analysing the structural dimension of the 'Corona Crisis' and precarity. In other words, questions of pandemics in the supposed conjunction with human rights will be looked at along the following lines.

- power
- knowledge
- caring for life
- escaping into living.

These issues are becoming in different contexts relevant; the fundamental line concerns the process of socialisation: in short, it must be said that we are confronted with aspects of the tension, subsequent to modernisation. While modern societies are characterised by a high degree of socialisation, occurring in a variety of forms, this is—seemingly a paradox—result of processes of individualisation. The immediate, 'peer-based' control as lower level of socialisation gains complexity in quantitative and qualitative terms, resulting from the increasing complexity of societal differentiation: while earlier critique of Niklas Luhmann's take on segmentary, social and functional differentiation is maintained *(see Herrmann, 1994),* it is now extended by way of interpreting the three forms of differentiation tangled in multiple ways: every main form of differentiation is at the very same time also interwoven with the two other forms which are themselves in multiple ways interwoven by the others. If we take functional differentiation as dominant form, this is itself also influenced by aspects of segmentary and social forms, while segmentary differentiation is also characterised by functional and social aspects and so on and so forth. We are here not confronted with a simultaneous occurrence but a close interlocking, each 'hinge' being the germ of a new social or sub-social speaking of 'social' in the understanding of the social quality approach).

Talking about responsibility is not least concerned with questions of property and the social obligation going hand in hand with it and the factual juxtaposition of social and individual. In the first case, social responsibility is (partially) approached independent of the principle that the party responsible is liable, and not only directed towards the social in general (e.g. the 'common weal') but also respecting 'individual others'; in other words, the point of departure of the definition is not located on the demand side but, instead, on the supply side. In the second case, such juxtaposition, supposedly a 'general' pattern, is in fact only valid under certain conditions of 'modernity'.

Precarity is then characterised by the growing gap between necessity and feasibility, while system maintenance has priority.

Talcott Parsons' notion of AGIL can help as it allows grasping the interplay between micro- and macro-level; however, it is by and large aiming on exploring an affirmative setting, not allowing understanding the tensions that are characterising processes of power-stricken socialisation, based on the principles of alienation and truncation.

Subsequently, it is suggested that power, knowledge, caring for life and escaping into living are also the lines along which precarity must be discussed. The principal pattern is a balance between different factors in the sense of an appropriate and accepted relation: a given distribution of power is accepted, not least on the basis of 'given and allowed' (conceded by the ruling classes) knowledge, making possible for individuals and classes/social strata alike to live in a satisfying way between self-determination and requirements by others/by the system.

In any case, such balance is temporary, its stability, sensitivity and exposure to factors that are fatal, destroying the actual system, replacing it by a new balance—however, during the interim phase we are witnessing a limbo. Rather than being *the best of times, the worst of times (Dickens),* it is a phase that can best be understood by using the words of Antonio Gramsci who contends that.

> the crisis consists precisely in the fact that the old is dying and the new cannot be born; in that interim period a great variety of morbid symptoms appear.' (Gramsci, 1930: 311; translation P.H.)

In short, the Corona crisis turns out to be a disclosure of the precarity of the current socio-political system, confronting societal actors on all levels with questioning the hitherto accepted system, the fundamental consensus—this time not by ideologies or different groups asking for the change of realities, but by changed realities demanding a new understanding thereof. Such different understanding is, however, not a matter of theory but an understanding of what must be done by whom and for whom. As such it is ultimately both, relational and self-enhancing. We find these processes on all three levels, i.e. the micro-, meso- and macro-level, thus resulting in a new analytical approach to precarity: it is the helplessness, or better: the inappropriateness of a socio-institutional system that lost its legitimation as consequence of the ultimate bond to use-value. In fact, it is a complex systemic disfunction, resulting from and feeding into divergence of three levels and two dimensions:

- micro- (i), meso- (ii) and macro (iii) level
  - (ad i) population at large and specific interest groups
  - (ad ii) political functionaries, polity
  - (ad iii) system—societal fabrique
- dimension of use value and exchange value.[3]

The new perspective on precarity can now be developed: first, we must differentiate between precarity and precariat. While it is in the meantime quite common to analyse the precariat, precarity is not an issue analysed as matter of structural weakness of socio-political processes of decision making. We define the precariat as a stratum: people with different class bonds, though knit together by the common position regarding labour: if (dis)integrated directly via the labour market or via self-employment/freelance activities, the socio-economic situation is characterised by 'enforced flexibility', i.e. the need to adapt to an open situation as far as the offer of work is concerned; and the quasi-unconditional acceptance of flexibility as far as the demand for labour is looked at, thus a closed situation in this respect. This means uncertainty, lack of ability to make plans (be it short term or long term), pressure on social and private relationships, often also decreasing readiness for and interest in an active lifestyle. These are some common features, applicable even if the material situation of concerned people may be extremely different. Talking about precarity, on the other hand, our interest is directed towards the increasing factual and objective alienation concerning the dimensions (ii) and (iii) from (i), also of (iii) from (ii). Simultaneously or not, we find alienation in respect of the dimensions, the exchange value becoming dominant. In simple terms we may say that increasing differentiation, as far as it is going hand in hand with specialisation, results in objective alienation which translates into truncation and the emergence of 'new' objectives, detached from what stands at the outset. Or again in other words: why should somebody—being functionary, i.e. functioning—in a high political or administrative position, feel any empathy about the real economy, i.e. the production and reproduction of every day's life. Instead, relevant is securing the system which is set on equal

---

[3] It is suggested that these 'dimensions', known from political economy, can—cum grano salis, and in application of the regulation theory, with the authors extension—also be applied when it comes to the analysis of political processes where political action is on the one hand immediately meaningful for (change of) the life regime and mode of living, while it is on the other hand relevant as 'positioning good'.

foot with securing the own position (or being promoted—what does it matter as long one agrees with David Graeber and his definition of bullshit jobs). Against this background the following analysis gains a distinct meaning: while the present analysis is on the one hand just a presentation of the politics, policies and polity, focussed on Germany, it provides on the other hand a narrative that allows a better understanding of the 'logic' behind the development. Becoming aware of the complex, not least historical, reasons behind today's political decisions under uncertainty and unpredictability, this may suggest some criteria for improving future policies. Bottom line is the presumption that

(i) human rights are on the definitional level characterised by tensions, depend-ing on the overall societal context, i.e. the overall context is the seedbed for the definition of something, and it does not matter if it is tensional or not: special attention must be paid to dimensions as individual-social; material-immaterial/ideal; responsibility of people-responsibility of institu-tions; responsibility for people-responsibility for institutions .... In this perspective it is difficult to know if a change of the balance sheet is needed: a major example during the pandemic's must be seen in effect that in highly individualised societies it is obviously difficult to oblige individuals to follow any rules, for instance accepting being vaccinated and wearing a protective masc. Important is to differentiate between people rejecting such measures as in their view the medical arguments concerning the usefulness of such measures is questionable and people rejecting such measures for 'principal reasons', simply because they refuse to accept any imposed obligation.— Thus, information, understood as enlightenment at its best, is a major point for consideration, bringing us to the second presumption, namely

(ii) the necessary relevance and consistency of polities, policies and politics—this is meant to refer to the 'internal consistency', i.e. the consistency of polities, policies and politics; but it refers also to cross-referential consistency, i.e. the consistency between the three areas.

In any case, one of the major problems is given by the fact that human rights have been initially claimed as protection against encroachments by the state. This is still a pattern standing in the background while being of utmost importance. At the same time, however, we see some changes in this pattern in two respects: on the one hand, the state is a highly differentiated institutional system, and the human rights issue is approached in different ways by the individual parts of this complex institutional system. On the other hand, there are other institu-tions with a quasi-statutory character and power, requiring that the protection of

Human Rights must be understood as well as protection against violations by non-statutory bodies. In any case, human rights must be seen not least as subject of power struggles.

The Pandemic—Also a Welcome Distraction

4

It is important to make from the outset clear that it is only possible to have a very limited view on what is going on or what had been going on in respect of Corona politics and policies. Many issues are necessarily faded out. It is important to underline this fact because it is easy to suggest arguments that have different emphasis or that are contradicting the thesis that will be put forward. For instance, the medical situation is not clear yet and it is definitely not clear in all the details. When it comes to political decisions the same is true with psychological effects on the side of the governed and the side of those who are governing; insecurity is also given if we look at the issue on the national level while we have—in particular in a multicentred era—limited insight into complex multinational developments, and even more so we have limited insight when it comes to assessing the impact at least as far as the global perspective is concerned.

The outline of the following is as follows: first there's the introduction, pointing out the complexity of the problem; the first main part, namely the presentation of the German political system, will present a look at the history of the state, its federalist structure and the changes; the second main part will present some main lines of policies concerned with the pandemics and the public perception; finally, some major issues will be raised, showing that policies mark their own way.

An entire range of issues—and in fact one of utmost importance – is by and large left out, namely the 'social question', the fact that the social position in society is a decisive factor especially when looking at the health issues around the Corona virus—its spread, its health impact, its treatment. Rupa Marya and Raj Patel ask their readers to

P. Herrmann, *Pandemics as Matter of a System Crisis,* Prekarisierung und soziale Entkopplung – transdisziplinäre Studien, https://doi.org/10.1007/978-3-658-43450-2_4

[r]ecall that in the Covid pandemic, not all patients had been equal. Shuffle through the X-rays from Covid-infected lungs, and you'll see a steady rhythm of overactivated immune response; look from bed to bed in an ICU filled with Covid patients, and you'll see patterns emerge. Black, Indigenous, and people of color (BIPOC) were overrepresented, their bodies subject to inflammation of all kinds, long before the SARS-CoV-2 virus ever settled into their lungs. Not only lack of access to health care, but systemic social and economic disenfranchisement rendered their bodies most susceptible to Covid when it hit. Their bodies were vulnerable and they were at risk for increased exposure to the virus due to the desperate need for an income and whether or not their work was deemed essential.(…) In California, 80 percent of undocumented workers were considered part of the 'essential critical infrastructure workforce' by the Department of Homeland Security.

(Marya/Patel, 2021: 10; cf. Eder, updated 17.05.2020-11:00)

This is in its own respect a crucially important and highly human-rights-relevant topic, by and large discussed under headings like social disadvantage/denial of social rights/social discrimination. But as important as these issues are, they still remain very much in the given framework, suggesting that in general terms society is in good order, only in need of some repair on the surface. The prevailing of such perspective is fact although over the last years an increasing awareness is coming to the fore, concerned with the finality of the capitalist system. Even a surely conservative writer as Frank Schirrmacher, for many years co-editor of the conservative FAZ hesitated, stating: *'Ich beginne zu glauben, dass die Linke recht hat' (I am beginning that the Left is right) (Schirrmacher, 2011)*. He continued by writing *'There are sentences that are wrong. And there are sentences that are right. It's bad when sentences that were wrong suddenly become right. Then the doubt about the overall rationality comes up. Then the doubts begin as to whether one has been right, throughout one's life.' (ibid.)* The core of his argument is not about policies—and failed (in the sense of malfunctioning and missed) intervention; while such critique plays a role, the real matter in question is

that neoliberalism [did not] come upon society like a brainwashing. It utilises the imaginative repository of bourgeois thinking: freedom, autonomy, self-determination with simultaneous respect for individual values, the chance to become who one wants to become, while at the same time taming the state and its omnipotence.

(ibid.)

As said, there will be only very limited reference made to these matters—the interest is, instead, directed to the general structural problems of the (German) polity, on the basis of which structural 'inequalities' evolve and that also lead to unjust policies and politics. This means, in turn, that any attempt to solve the 'social problems' has to consider the fundamental character of the challenge, accepting that there are surely measures needed to immediately overcome social injustice and hardships where possible, nevertheless, the long term challenge is one that has to consider the precarious character of a mode of socialisation (or here: polity), that is based on and geared to limited spaces (nation states and its subunits) whereas the matters that require attention are going far beyond and need in fact attention beyond any borders, be it spatial, temporal and social.

Limitations: Decision Making Under the Condition of Uncertainty and with Limited Knowledge

5

As said, there are many aspects and we can only deal with one at a time—this makes it especially problematic or difficult for any political system taking up challenges during a period of pandemics, not least because there is at least for a more or less long initial phase not sufficient knowledge about the medical and virological aspects, the prospects regarding the duration of the problem cannot be made out, and the behaviour of people may hugely vary. Of course, every political system must build on or must deal with something that is difficult to predict—a truism at any time; however, these exceptional situations, phases or eras[1] mean that we are confronted with the necessity to take decisions under conditions of uncertainty or even worse, of not knowing the consequences of our action at all, being forced to accept the Rumsfeld-notion of *'the unknown unknowns'*. This is even more complicated because the consequences are not limited to just one area but spreading in the extreme case globally: we have the medical issues, we have the political issues in the area of politics, we are dealing with policies, we have the topics of rights, of legitimacy, of long-term responsibility and unclear liability and sets of complex long-term obligations.[2] It has to be considered as

---

[1] Frequently the term *turning point in history* is used these days.

[2] In general, state liability is subordinate always subject to the principle of the party responsible being liable to pay and the principle of individual responsible. Thus, it is Aufgabe des Staatshaftungsrechts, einen Ausgleich zugunsten derjenigen vorzusehen, die durch schuldhaftes, vor allem aber auch durch rechtswidriges Handeln von Amtsträgern einen Schaden erlitten haben. (Becker, 2018: 90). This reflects not least what will be said when it comes later to the discussion of 'dignity', where we will find the question of state responsibility left

P. Herrmann, *Pandemics as Matter of a System Crisis,* Prekarisierung und soziale Entkopplung – transdisziplinäre Studien, https://doi.org/10.1007/978-3-658-43450-2_5

well that parts of what happens today, of what governments decide—and ignore—
is (almost) necessarily following from the political system, here the polity and its
history in Germany: path-dependency is a complex relationality in its own short-
and long-term processuality.

---

open to the state withdrawing from responsibility, in favour of the right of the individual to
non-intervention.

The Constitutional State Without Constitution

6

The underlying thesis of this contribution is that we are dealing with a constitutional state without a constitution—at least up to the so-called unification this is without any doubt true although too often not recognised. We find the official statement, clearly marking the conscious and intended delay of a constitution for the state of West Germany. The background of this decision is going back to the original intention, clearly stated in the Basic Law of the zones occupied by the Allied Western powers: from the Western perspective, two states of German nation[1] had only been accepted for a transition period, and the GDR had not been officially acknowledged as independent, sovereign state. The Western powers aimed on having one German state at some stage, having a 'unified' Germany again and it must be said that this had been undoubtedly a decision maintained under the aegis of the former FRG, the western part of Germany until 1989, then

---

[1] In fact, Western Germany did not consider the GDR as state, and—related—saw itself as fragment, Carlo Schmid contending that the relevant body—after lively debate—agreed '*to a large extent with my considerations, according to which a constitution for a state in West Germany should not be established, but only an organisational statute for an administrative area of West Germany encompassing the three zones. This organisational statute should be called the Basic Law and should not be adopted by a constituent assembly, but by a parliamentary council to be appointed by the Land parliaments of the Länder.*' (Schmid, 1981: 329; Translation P.H.) In principle, this is true also for the GDR—while there had been a 'proper constitution' in place, this went for a long time hand in hand with the assumption of unification at some stage. The final solution of the question of the 'sustainability' of the state had to wait until the takeover of the GDR by the FRG, in some way combined with the attempt to deny the existence of the GDR as part of German history (see e.g. Emmerich, 2010).

P. Herrmann, *Pandemics as Matter of a System Crisis,* Prekarisierung und soziale Entkopplung – transdisziplinäre Studien, https://doi.org/10.1007/978-3-658-43450-2_6

suggesting that *what belongs together grows together.*[2] All this meant as well that the relevant actors had been clearly saying and claiming that unification would only be possible under capitalist conditions. The German Basic Law consequently states:

> *This Basic Law shall cease to be valid on the day on which a constitution comes into force which has been freely decided by the German people.*

Before engaging in detail of what this means, some aspects must be pointed out, even today still linked to the process of 'unification' and the [cl]aim of Germany having finally a constitution. An official statement of the German government states the following:

> *On 1 July 1948, the military governors of the British, French and American occupation zones instructed the prime ministers of the West German Länder to have a constitution drawn up.*
>
> *On 23 May 1949, the Basic Law was finally solemnly promulgated and signed in Bonn. It came into force the following day.*
>
> *Initially not for the whole nation*
>
> *The term 'constitution' was deliberately avoided: The Basic Law did not constitute a constitution for the entire German people, nor did full sovereignty prevail in its area of application. It was intended to be an interim solution until an all-German constitution could be established.*
>
> *This interim solution was also expressed in the preamble ('for a transitional period') and in the final article 146: 'This Basic Law shall cease to be valid on the day on which a constitution comes into force which has been freely decided by the German people.*
>
> *With the completion of the unification of Germany on 3 October 1990, the Basic Law became the constitution of the whole of Germany.*
>
> (https://www.bundesregierung.de/breg-de/themen/grundgesetz-fuer-die-bundesrep ublik-deutschland-454028; 05.06.21)

Looking at the events in preparation of the unification, the follow-up, the execution and again the follow-up, there is no clear evidence of a peoples' decision, a plebiscite that actually had been set as precondition for changing the German *Grundgesetz,* the Basic Law, into a constitution. Of course, there is not any point

---

[2] Willy Brandt said this with reference to the two German states, though he actually referred to Europe *(see* https://www.dw.com/de/willy-brandt-es-wächst-zusammen-was-zusammen-gehört/a-16431107; 02/09/2023).

in bringing this to the constitutional court, questioning what is now the German constitution; nevertheless, we have to acknowledge that in actual fact the so-called unification had been a process happening behind the scene, undermining what the people, many people at least, wanted.

Furthermore, the unification and the state of the specifically defined constitution did have, indeed, also very important international dimensions: the fact of regulating the entire matter with concluding the *Treaty on the Final Settlement with Respect to Germany (German: Vertrag über die abschließende Regelung in Bezug auf Deutschland)*, is of major importance not least in respect of certain dimension of the liability. A strict legally oriented argumentation may at first glance suggest that the FRG, as it is currently defined, can justifiably refrain for instance from paying back the 'loan' (forced loan) received from Greece—the said two-plus-four-agreement.[3]

> was intended by the Allies to settle all outstanding questions concerning Germany and to take the place of a formal peace treaty. It is true that the document is silent on the issue of reparations, and usually matters not included in a treaty are not supposed to be settled. At the time, however, it was precisely the intention of the contracting parties to settle all outstanding issues with the treaty. A silence therefore does have explanatory value—namely that the London moratorium is to be continued, i.e. that no further reparation payments are outstanding.
>
> (Fenrich, 2015; translation P.H.])

Of special relevance in the present context is the fact that the entire German polity is geared to establish a hegemonial system—nationally and internationally. So Katrin Fenrich continues that

> [t]he real problem is Greece's lack of participation in the Two-Plus-Four Treaty. If one interprets the treaty as a waiver of all possibly outstanding reparation claims, it would be a treaty to the detriment of third parties, since Greece, as a non-contracting party, would have its rights curtailed.
>
> (ibid.)

All this does not suggest that a continuation of the constellation of the German states before '89 would have been an option, but it would at least question the path it took—many people from a very different political backgrounds consider *this* unification for good reasons as takeover.

---

[3] Interestingly, the German name speaks of a Vertrag (treaty/contract) whereas the English name says agreement.

Decisively, the role of law is seen as central element of the basic law, and thus of this new state, obviously not least as answer to fascism—the historical background against which it emerged. Having said this, there had been in the early years of the FRG or West Germany—or the three western zones—a fierce debate on the way of the development after fascism. One important point must be seen in the fact that the Christian Democrats, already then a conservative party, standing against the Social Democrats—at that time shifting already towards people's party[4]— announced in their Ahlener program the following:

> *The capitalist economic system has not done justice to the state and social life interests of the German people. After the terrible political, economic and social collapse as a result of criminal power politics, only a reorganisation from the bottom up can take place. The content and aim of this social and economic reorganisation can be no more than the capitalist striving for profit and power, but only the well-being of our people. Through a public economic order, the German people shall receive an economic and social constitution which corresponds to the right and dignity of man, serves the spiritual and material development of our people and secures internal and external peace.*
>
> *(CDU, 1947)*[5]

With this, the CDU was aiming at least verbally on a socialist strategy. So, while it had been on the one hand clear that the new state would be a *Rechtsstaat,* a state based on law, or: a constitutional state, it had been equally clear that there have been different political strengths, different strategies in the political debate, put forward by different forces. The one can be characterised as authoritarian rule, defining the state as central power. While it had been thought of as constitutional state, it had been at the same time with an exceptionally strong executive. Historically, it had been or still is known under the term of the *Obrigkeitsstaat,* an authoritarian state, with the unquestionable superior power of the government and in particular its executive—one could also speak of a Machiavellian state for which achieving a specific purpose is the highest good whereas ethical considerations are seen as potential tool, arbitrarily used or ignored, depending on the given circumstances. Being decisive when it came to decisions of the political structure and the distribution of power, there had been a strong emphasis on the need of regulation—the consideration of what should be regulated and who had been seen as regulating and regulated subjects. Emmerich contends—interestingly for both German states:

---

[4] Later laid down in their Godesberg program.

[5] Of course, detailed reading quickly shows that this had been a veil for a 'new capitalism'.

It is obviously part of the traditions in this country that the German people need either God, Emperor, Tribune, or at least a head. Already in the Paulskirche constitution of 1849 it had said: 'The head of the empire bears the title: Emperor of the Germans. The person of the Emperor is inviolable'.

(Emmerich, 2010: 41 f.; translation P.H.)

However, there had been different interpretations, one not least emphasising an abstract spirit of freedom—in particular individual freedom and freedom of the market—positioning this as superior idea over any other consideration, thus presenting an ideology standing against the fact of the superiority of the executive. It had been as well interesting that on the one hand the Christian Democrats emphasized a 'socialist strategy', while the so-called social market economy had been centre-staged under Ludwig Erhardt, minister for economic affairs from 1949–1963. Leaving other interesting aspects aside, e.g. the half-hearted policy of competition control, the interesting point for the present discussion is given by the fact that the roots of this program can be located in the catholic social teaching and its foundation of the principle of subsidiarity, emphasising the responsibility of the 'smallest unit', namely the individual and his/her family *(see Pope Leo XIII, 1891; Pope Pius XI, 1931)*, the latter stating in paragraph 79

And when we speak of the reform of institutions, we think first of the state, not because all salvation is to be expected from its work, but because, because of the vice of individualism, as we have said, things are reduced to such a point that, having demolished and almost extinguished the ancient rich form of social life, which once took place through a complex of different associations, individuals and the state are left almost alone. And such a deformation of the social order does no small damage to the state itself, on which all the burdens fall, which those destroyed corporations can no longer bear, and which finds itself burdened with an infinity of burdens and affairs.

(Pope Pius XI, 1931: para 79)

In other words, it had been about the responsibility of everybody for him/herself, from there building up different layers, leaving the central state or any superordinated power only stepping in as a supportive mechanism. The latter had been later interpreted by Nell-Breuning as obligation of the superordinate levels to secure the frame for action, in his words:

The principle proclaims the help of the community for its members as a 'duty' ('subsidiarium officium'!) and demands that this help should really be real help, helpful help, should not patronise or incapacitate the member, but should rather help him or her to fully develop his or her God-given talents and powers, and therefore the help should be as much as possible help for self-help. The so-called 'right of small circles of life' is derived from this as a rule of responsibility: What the narrower and therefore closer circle of life can do for its members, the wider and higher circle of life (the 'higher authority') should not take away from it, but leave to it and help it, because in this way the member in need of help is enabled to participate more, not so much outside help as the maximum amount of help for self-help is granted.

(Nell-Breuning, 1.3.1986; translated P.H.)

We should indeed ask—for instance with Hermann Klenner *(see Klenner, 2009: 11–15)* – why the sovereignty of the state is still not meant to be sovereignty of the people. Here is exactly the point made by Schirrmacher—as quoted earlier— namely the ambiguity that comes at a certain historical point to the fore, making a pronounced conservative intellectual asking if the left is right.

From 'Social Contract' to Contract Society

7

While in debates on the catholic teaching the aspect of solidarity is frequently emphasised, it can be said that structurally individualism had been centre-staged.

This had been backed by and translated into the emphasis of the legal system and its inherent binary code—the limitation had been frequently highlighted as for instance in general terms by Niklas Luhmann and his works on general media and autopoiesis, the application of systems theory by sociology of law in Gunther Teubner's reflections and the importance of extra-legal reflections standing behind social law as emphasised by Hans-F. Zacher. The very core of the autopoietic take on law is given by the fact that law remains caught in its own reflection. Justice had been reduced on legality and legality on contractual relationships between— natural or legal—personalities. This had been always considered to be a question of individual decisions and moreover as standard used to guide decisions. In other words, assessing contracts is by definition a matter of individual approaches to justice—one has to hesitate to use the term justice because, as said, justice is reduced on legality, substantially discharged as already outlined in Immanuel Kant's short essay *Ueber ein Vermeintes Recht aus Menschenliebe zu luegen.* As Kant states

A lie, then, defined merely as a deliberately untrue declaration against another person, does not need the addition that it must harm another; as the jurists demand for its definition (mendacium est falsiloquium in praeiudicium alterius). For it always harms another, if not another man, yet humanity in general, by making the source of law useless.

(Kant, 1779 ; translation P.H.)

P. Herrmann, *Pandemics as Matter of a System Crisis,* Prekarisierung und soziale Entkopplung – transdisziplinäre Studien, https://doi.org/10.1007/978-3-658-43450-2_7

The quote is only seemingly distant from the analysis of the present polity analysis. It clearly shows that even the state is in last instance 'individualised' as actor. It must be emphasised that this statement does not aim on discrediting law. However, we should understand this legal system is structurally limited and has shortcomings.

Competition Society—the State of Law as State of the Fittest

This had been necessarily a double-edged sword, ending in a socio-economic system that had been moving towards a three pillar system, based on employment and welfare states, a growth-dependency of the entire security system (otherwise this economic system would not be able to prevail) and with this of course a strong export strategy on which the entire system had been built (otherwise it would not have been possible to move towards such strategy, not internally and let alone globally). These had been conditions for a political institutional system, implying a hierarchically ordered polity, moving economically towards an export-based growth-strategy, of which the social (security) system had been depending on full-employment; this (up to some point clandestine) rebirth of an expansionist strategy had been a strong factor, determining 'national identity'. The centrality of these arrays meant in many cases as well federal responsibility *(see Basic Law, current version, articles 70 ff., 91 a-c, e; qualifying 23, 24, 32)*. While this leaves seemingly many areas to the Laender, the federal level functions factually in several ways as 'superpower': a growing number of competencies had been attributed to the federal level, compensated for by an increasing co-determination by the federal council (upper house of the parliament); in addition, the financial structure is also characterised by a strong tendency to centralism. This is important as in the public opinion as well as factually the federal structure is at least blurred and of lesser importance. On the other hand, it means that the Laender tend in many cases to look for opportunities to raise their image.

Importantly, the finance, industrial and economic policies (and with this the area of employment) are dominated by the federal level. At the end, one decisive

P. Herrmann, *Pandemics as Matter of a System Crisis,* Prekarisierung und soziale Entkopplung – transdisziplinäre Studien, https://doi.org/10.1007/978-3-658-43450-2_8

37

problem of the entire federalist structure in Germany—and this is of central meaning when we will later discuss concrete policies dealing with the pandemics—is given by the way of financing that leaves the Lander and even more so the Municipalities standing in the rain.

Finally, the approach to federalism had been in actual fact a pragmatic way of a new form of establishing superpower, claiming that equality and mutual recognition would prevail instead of a global dimension as a newly emerging world power. Again, we see the importance of the geopolitical dimension of the entire debate. This can be briefly captured by four aspects. First, we are dealing with a divided and possibly even multiple-divided country, having the two different German states and having in in addition the occupational powers, dividing the FRG into different zones, meaningful not only during the first years after the war, but actually in a long-term perspective, unconsciously characterising in different ways the concerned Laender. We have at the same time a somewhat consolidated system of the two states (FRG and GDR), at least for some time coexisting without any real efforts towards unification; however, and second, it is important to keep in mind, that it had been always the underlying and outspoken aim of the Western powers to have sole and complete control over the German nation—laid out in article 23 of the Basic Law—in its original formulation it reads as followed

For the time being, this Basic Law shall apply in the territory of the Laender Baden, Bavaria, Bremen, Greater Berlin, Hamburg, Hesse, Lower Saxony, North Rhine-Westphalia, Rhineland-Palatinate, SchleswigHolstein, Wuerttemberg-Baden and Wuerttemberg-Hohenzollern. It shall be put into force for other parts of Germany on their accession.

This had been complemented by article 146, contending

This Basic Law shall become invalid on the day when a constitution adopted in a free decision by the German people comes into force.

Third, federalism had been of course a conscious strategy, but it had been as well a strategy, guided by a pragmatic approach because of the multiple powers involved (the four occupying allied forces and the various groups in Germany), all playing a role with their different strategies. While it is not necessary to take up the entire debate on federalism and it's philosophy, as it can be seen for instance in *The Federalist Papers* in the United States of Northern America, the approach had been in the German post WW-II-case more pragmatic, clearly expressed in the conference of the six nations, namely the United States of Northern America,

France, Great Britain and the Benelux-countries and excluding the Soviet Union, coming to the following definition or decision about the future of the German state: they

> *recognise, taking into account in the present situation, that it is necessary to give the German people the opportunity to achieve, on the basis of free and democratic form of government, the eventual re-establishment of German unity, at present disrupted. In these circumstances they have reached the conclusion that it would be desirable that the German people in the different States should now be free to establish for themselves the political organization and institutions which will enable them to assume those governmental responsibilities which are compatible with the minimum requirements of occupation and control and which ultimately will enable them to assume full governmental responsibility. Then delegates consider that the people in the States will wish to establish a constitution with provisions which will allow all the German States to subscribe a soon as circumstances permit.*

> *Therefore the delegates have agreed to recommend to their Governments that the Military Governors should hold a joint meeting with the Ministers-President of the Western zone in Germany. At this meeting the Ministers-President will be authorized to convene a Constituent Assembly in order to prepare a Constitution for the approval of the participating States.*

> *Delegates to this Constituent Assembly will be chosen in each of the States I accordance with procedure and regulations to be determined by the legislative bodies in the individual States. The Constitution should be such as to enable the Germans to play their part in bringing to an end the present division of Germany, not by the reconstitution of a centralized Reich nut by means f a federal form of government which adequately protects the rights of the respective States, and which at the same time provides for adequate central authority and which guarantees the rights and freedoms of the individual.*

> *If the Constitution as prepared by the Constituent Assembly does not conflict with these general principles, the Military Governors will authorize its submissions for ratification by the people in the respective States.*

(Text 1948)

A diffuse practical reasoning behind the federalist approach after the second world war and fascism, standing clearly against a centralist system, and going hand in hand with a firm and dangerous confrontation with the USSR and the eastern part of Germany that became in October 1949 the GDR, four days after the foundation of the FRG, can be taken as another way of capturing the constellation. The statement by James K. Pollock, US-advisor, shows how strong this confrontational course had been:

> *But make no mistake about it, when we go that far and when we make a political*
> *amalgamation of western Germany as against eastern Germany, then we had better*
> *dig in and prepare for what seems to me to be the inevitable conflict which will come*
> *sooner or later. We have then drawn the line between the East and West in such an*
> *irretrievable and unchangeable fashion that we will immediately be thrown into the*
> *possibility of a conflict.*
>
> *(Pollock, June 9, 1947)*

Fourth, then, whatever had been said and still must be said about fascism, its roots and traditions in Germany, it has to be said as well that there was a clear movement against this kind of centralist principle. The motivation behind the different notions and demands had been definitely different, each of the relevant powers having a distinct ideological and strategic take. In fact there had been already some form of federalism in place, at least suggesting a path-dependency beyond the tradition of the German Laender; one aspect is given by the constellation of two states of German nationality (the Western powers, in particular the powers in Western Germany never fully acknowledging the GDR as independent and sovereign state, always claiming the superior meaning of nationhood over statehood); another point is given by the 'independence movement' for instance in Bavaria and the Bavarian leg of the Cristian democrats, insisting on its independence in the 'Free State of Bavaria', moreover, the Bavarian parliament even not voting in favour of the German Basic law[1]; furthermore the special status of the Saarland with its short, though changeable history, joining the FRG only in 1955; and finally the fact of feeling a kind of guilt on the side of the different powers, pushing them to search for a political system that could secure pan-German capitalism and the pan-German political power at least in the territory of the FRG, avoiding the re-emergence of a German superpower,[2] while within

---

[1] As the majority of the Laender voted in favour of it, it had been also legally valid in the 'free state'—see article 144 of the Basic Law, in its original version of 1949.

[2] The communique of the six-power London conference stating.

> It was affirmed that Germany must not again be permitted to become an aggressive power and that prior to the general withdrawal of the forces of occupation agreement will be reached among the Governments concerned with respect to necessary measures of demilitarization, disarmament and control of industry and with respect to occupation of key areas. Also there should be a system of inspection to ensure to maintenance of the agreed provisions of German disarmament and demilitarization. (Text 1948)

the FRG there had been, of course, the strive for independence from the powers within the Western occupational zones and later FRG. At the end we see a kind of compromise, declared at the end of the London Six-Power Conference, and already quoted earlier.

A long and winded road—all this may seem to be off topic. However, we need a sound understanding of those patterns that stand economically, juridically and in terms of polities behind what I suggest to be a contemporary anthropology of law and politics. Only knowing the roots, allows us to know the leaves and blossoms, and this way we may also find cures if needed.

Motherly Encouragement: We Can Do It!   9

Probably, Mutti Merkel—mammy Merkel—is by now well-known beyond the German borders as nickname of the former German chancellor: a somewhat affectionate, disrespectful, dismissive characterisation of a lady of whom one cannot be sure if she is naïve and compassionate, pragmatic, sober and calculating in the spirit of her professional training in physics, strategically ruthless, shrewd and power-obsessed or some kind of mixture and merger of these characteristics.

In a way, the wording during a press conference in March 2020 is telling:

Our solidarity, our reason and our heart for each other are already being put to the test, and I hope that we will also pass this test.

(Merkel, 11.03.2020)

Admittedly, it is easy to criticise policies in an exceptional situation as we faced it since the outbreak of the pandemics. The policies and the analyses are even more difficult if we consider that in addition to path-dependency in such a situation three facts make the situation even more difficult: first, every step determines the next—a common pattern of policy making, however having more weight in such crises-situation; second, daily policymaking on the verge of a state of emergency is by definition facing exceptional challenges in terms of legitimation; third, not least, *the show must go on though the spotlight changed completely,* or in a more sober formulation: pandemics and related measures overshadowed everything else, not allowing that anything else would be discharged from dealing with its own genuine topics.

© The Author(s), under exclusive license to Springer Fachmedien Wiesbaden   43
GmbH, part of Springer Nature 2023
P. Herrmann, *Pandemics as Matter of a System Crisis,* Prekarisierung und soziale
Entkopplung – transdisziplinäre Studien,
https://doi.org/10.1007/978-3-658-43450-2_9

One can say that initially the danger of the virus had not been understood. Although its existence had not been denied, the severeness of the intrusion had not been recognised immediately. Even the controls at the national borders had been as relaxed as usual, no special care being taken. While the danger had been seen in general terms, it had been often met with an attitude of denial of personal and national relevance. While we saw on the one hand some forms of blaming China, it had been perhaps even with a kind of gloating, not accepting notion that the virus would not know any borders. Telling is the title page of *Der Spiegel,* presenting its 1st February 2020-edition with a rebuke of China, manipulatively suggesting China 'going to war with the virus', while in some way also acknowledging that the problem is not China, but one of geopolitics.

Leaving the multitude of reasons and perhaps reasoning aside, one important aspect is given by the historical experience of the post-WW-II-years, witnessing long-term positive development of the entire social system, including the health sector, in the FRG. While there is no straightforward answer, it is at the end of the day the federal level, signing responsible for the health sector, although much of the financial burden is left on the shoulders of the decentral level (Laender and even municipalities). The latter means that we are confronted with a major tension that had been for several years veiled by relative success and the global constellation. However, already since some time these conditions of success had been undermined—the so-called Laenderfinanzausgleich ('fiscal equalisation revenue') did not provide sufficient resources, the increasing role of the pharmaceutical-technical complex increased the expenses, the demographic development required more investment; the financialisation and underlying orientation on cost-effectiveness (and even profitability) contributed in different ways to the decreasing quality and especially nationally comprehensive supply especially with emergency beds and equipment. Under conditions of pandemics this translated into another meaning of emergency in connection with the health care system. It became also obvious that the income and working conditions of hospital staff had been visibly problematic: increased requirements could not be answered and in particular staff in the public sector had been working up to their limits, but also making the misery of the medical and care sector obvious. We can also see a time gap: while these developments took already during the last Kohl-government shape, they came to full consciousness only much later— not least due to the coincidence of multiple crises, amongst others the global finance crisis,[1] decreasing purchasing power effecting many social strata while the gap between the rich and poor increased, the skyrocketing increase of cost

---

[1] Not least putting the German system of universal banking under additional pressure.

for accommodation. Importantly, and this seems to be a global trend, the 'social question', traditionally attributed to the working class, is now reaching out into the middle class and the younger generation. The widespread expectation, that the young generation would be better-off than their parents, is by and large factually questioned. Decisively, under these conditions the suitability of the federal polity reached objectively its limits and the legitimacy of the polity and specifically the process of unification came under major pressure.

Answers given under pressure are usually not well chosen. A major benefit is given by the—though contradictory—reputation by Mutti Merkel and her pragmatic approach. In fact, this, together with the 'federal mess', allowed her, the central government and the heads of the Laender-governments to pursue for probably about half of the period between the first acknowledgment and mid-2021 a by and large unquestioned 'soft authoritarian rule'. Three main pillars can be seen.

First, we must mention the quasi-objectivation by establishing an expertocratic link to one institute with specific expertise (Robert-Koch-Institute and one virologist, namely Christian Drosten)—although experts, including Drosten, emphasised the need of *political* decisions, for which they would only provide data, this expertise had been used as a kind of thought-terminating cliché. Angela Merkel, on the occasion of a press conference on the 11th of March 2020 stated.

> the standards for our actions, our political actions, are derived from what scientists and experts tell us. That is why it is also very important to me that not only the Federal Minister of Health is sitting here with me today, but also the institute that stands for this expertise, together with many proven experts, namely the Robert Koch Institute and its head, Professor Wieler.
>
> (Merkel, 11.03.2020 :edited; translated, P.H.)

Second, meetings between chancellor and heads of the Laender had been the central decision-making instance which can be seen for two reasons as problematic.

(i) Decisions had been taken without the needed parliamentarian backing—this is at least one possible interpretation. Most relevant are the *Basic Law* on the one hand and most fundamental, the *Gesetz zur Verhütung und Bekämpfung von Infektionskrankheiten beim Menschen (Infektionsschutzgesetz—IfSG)*, i.e. the *Law on the Prevention and Control of Infectious Diseases in Humans (Protection against Infection Act—IfSG)* (https://www.gesetze-im-internet.de/ifsg/index.html; 18/06/2021). It may come as a surprise, that it had been—legally backed by Art. 74 Abs. 1 Nr. 19, Art. 72 Abs. 1 GG—only issued on the 20th of June 2020, enacted on the 1st of January 2021, completely replacing the *Gesetz zur Verhütung und Bekämpfung übertragbarer Krankheiten beim Menschen (Act on the Prevention and Control of Communicable Diseases in Humans)* from 1961. Interestingly it is part of 'general administrative law'.

Not applicable are the so-called *Notstandsgesetze ('Emergency Acts')*, a term used for the *17th amendment of the Basic Law.*[2] The inclusion of such clause (in fact: changes of some articles) had been condition, set by the Allied Occupational Forces, insisting on such regulation. Such inclusion had been somewhat paradoxical as the quest had been given by the wish to have the occupying troops protected by the (Western) German state, on the other hand the promise to withdraw the troops and grant full sovereignty under the condition of such regulation. In short, the pandemics constituted in legal terms at most a quasi-emergency, as such not allowing recurs on the 'emergency act '.

(ii) These meetings had also been used as stage to improve the image of individuals and the represented county, while the chancellor used this as platform to push her own ideas through. The most remarkable case occurred when during one of the meetings a decision had been taken regarding a lock-down in particular for Maundy-Thursday. Merkel recalled it a short time after the decision had been taken and proclaimed, taking full personal responsibility.

Dr Angela Merkel, Federal Chancellor: Mr President, colleagues! Ladies and Gentlemen! Today I informed the Minister Presidents of the Länder and the chairpersons of the parliamentary groups of the German Bundestag, and subsequently also the public, that I decided this morning not to initiate the necessary regulations for the additional so-called Easter rest, i.e. the days of on Maundy Thursday and Holy Saturday, but to stop them.....

This mistake is solely mine; because in the end I bear the ultimate responsibility for everything—that is qua office—(Beatrix von Storch [AfD]: Then draw the consequence!) so also for the decision taken on Monday for the so-called Easter rest. A mistake must be named to be a mistake, above all it must be corrected, and if possible, this must be done in good time. (Applause from the CDU/CSU and members of the SPD) Nevertheless, I am of course aware that this entire process has caused additional uncertainty. I deeply regret this, and I would like to take this opportunity to apologise once again to the citizens and also to you, ladies and gentlemen. (Beatrix von Storch [AfD]: No!) I regret this additional uncertainty all the more because—unfortunately— we are in the middle of the third wave of the pandemic, which has been triggered so severely by the mutations.

(Merkel, 24.3.2021; translation P.H.)

---

[2] Of special relevance Basic Law, articles 10, 20.4, 35, 115.

Then, continuing:

> *The pandemic has hit our society painfully on some key points. .... . It also affects our society's self-image. In this self-image, such an event as this pandemic was actually no longer foreseen. It actually contradicts our concept of security, of health, of advanced medicine and medical technology. It also contradicts our expectations of the community, of the state, that health care will work and can be guaranteed. Illness has been an individual problem in these advanced societies, but it has not been a social or even a political problem.*

(*ibid.*)

The general notion of living in a performance and competition society had now been complemented by the notion of a society of distrust. After the questionable promise of 'blossoming landscapes'[3] as result of the so-called unification, the pandemic confronted the population another time with promises turning out as questionable: the assurance of socio-physical security, guaranteed by a well-developed and expensive social insurance and the reality of a health threat for which nobody would sign responsible, on the contrary: governments and businesses feeling themselves uncomfortably threatened, while the quest for responsible actors increased. An attitude of fear, panic, egoism and egocentrism continued in one way or another—the mindset itself did not change, only the framework changed, leading to even more pronounced expressions. The fact of the structural character of failures and contradictions became obvious in various ways—not least by the opposition equally lacking constructivist proposals.

Urgent issues are highlighted in the following:

(i)   the legitimation of the chancellor to recall without democratic legitimation a decision that had been taken by a political body that lacked itself full democratic legitimation;

(ii)   Merkel's statement during a talk show on the 28th of March 2021, that she would insist on hard measures *(*https://www.ndr.de/nachrichten/info/Angela-Merkel-zu-Gast-bei-Anne-Will,audio860140.html*; 18/06/2021;* https://youtu.be/UpEPnbgPkm0*; 19/06/2021);*

---

[3] Kohl, then Chancellor the 'new Germany' contended „Durch eine gemeinsame Anstrengung wird es uns gelingen, Mecklenburg/Vorpommern und Sachsen-Anhalt, Brandenburg, Sachsen und Thüringen schon bald wieder in blühende Landschaften zu verwandeln, in denen es sich zu leben und zu arbeiten lohnt.' (Kohl, 1990).

(iii) the 'democratically precarious dimension' of the decision of the German Parliament concerning the *Gesetzesbeschluss des Deutschen Bundestages Viertes Gesetz zum Schutz der Bevölkerung bei einer epidemischen Lage von nationaler Tragweite (Bundesrat Drucksache 315/21; 21.04.2021;* https://www.bundesrat.de/SharedDocs/drucksachen/2021/0301-0400/315-21.pdf?__blob=publicationFile&v=1; *13/07/2021),* which may be seen as kind of enabling act, transferring unprecedented powers to the Federal Level;

(iv) the fact that already earlier far-reaching power had been transferred to the federal level, for instance in the 'Social Protection Package' *(Deutscher Bundestag Drucksache 19/18107 19. Wahlperiode 24.03.2020 Gesetzentwurf der Fraktionen der CDU/CSU und SPD Entwurf eines Gesetzes für den erleichterten Zugang zu sozialer Sicherung und zum Einsatz und zur Absicherung sozialer Dienstleister aufgrund des Coronavirus SARS-CoV-2 (Sozialschutz-Paket);* https://dserver.bundestag.de/btd/19/181/1918107.pdf; *10.07.2021—bill in favour of easier access to social security and on the use and protection of social services providers due to the SARS-CoV-2 Coronavirus),* changing § 67 SGB II, allowing to take decisions without hearing the Parliament of the Laender and stating in § 5 *The Federal Government is authorised to extend the special guarantee mandate by statutory order without the consent of the Bundesrat until a date beyond 30 September 2020, but no later than 31 December 2020..'* (https://www.bundesrat.de/SharedDocs/drucksachen/2021/0301-0400/315-21.pdf?__blob=publicationFile&v=1; *13/07/2021; translation P.H.);*

(v) finally, it became known that recalling the decision had not least been consequence of strong lobbying activities—and this raises the general question to which extent it had been the RKI, the government as democratically elected instance or strong interest groups that dominated political decisions.

This must be seen as well against a wider background—shedding some light on potential dysfunctions of a federalist polity with unclear profile and blurred competencies as it had been outlined throughout the text earlier. If and to the extent to which it is true that the German polity structurally lacks clarity, it is also clear that it is not least used as stage for competition between persons/candidates. Is it completely overstretching this point, making reference to Machiavelli and his remark at the end of the 5th chapter of *Il Principe?* There we read

> *But when the cities or provinces are used to live under a prince, and that blood is extinguished, since they are used to obeying on the one hand, and on the other not*

*having an old prince, they do not agree to make one between them, they do not know
how to live free; so that they are later to take up arms, and it is easier for a prince
to gain and ensure their freedom. But in the public kingdoms there is more life, more
hatred, more desire for vengeance; nor can the memory of ancient liberty let them rest:
such that the surest way is to extinguish them or inhabit them.*

(Machiavelli, 1632: 17; translation P.H.)

For several times, the especially the Bavarian minister president engaged in a
way—and thus provoked the chancellor to engage equally—that the impression
that power games are more important than pandemic issues were not unlikely,
given that the Federal elections were issued for September 2021.

Third, and in some ways crosscutting, the acceptance of major contradictions
and inconsistencies—one extreme case had been the obligation to wear masks
in the Deutsche Bahn (German railway) during the early phase. As it had been
at that time Laender-Sache, i.e. a matter to be decided on the decentral level,
people had to wear the protective mask or not, depending on the location of the
train—it happened that there had been different rules during one and the same
trip, in other words: one could take-off the mask/had to use it, depending on
where, in which of the counties, the train travelled—and of course, provided one
would be aware of the train having crossed a border. While this had been surely
an extreme case, the various inconsistencies contributed to an increasing number
of cases where people approached the implementation of the requirements in a
more or less relaxed, not to say: they had been ignored. This, on the other hand,
evoked in some cases harsh measures by the police. It can be debated if such
interventions had been politically motivated, directed against political rallies of
any kind or if it had been an expression of the helplessness of the police forces
(be it the individual guards, the units or the command centres).

One of the decisive problematiques is given by the fact of a completely
inscrutable and incomprehensible set of rules and ruling. Merkel's apologies
marked indeed in various respects a kind of turning point: (i) It concerned a
major decision—and the turn caused a major general turn and also threat on
the remaining legitimacy, the statement can then be seen as the government and
the chancellor crawling before the people. (ii) It had also been a phase that can
be characterised by a turn of the public opinion—yes, weather matters and the
looming spring made living under the conditions of lockdown more difficult. In
fact, there is a complex jigsaw as for instance outdoor life is for many at least in
part an escape from miserable housing conditions. (iii) Not least, it had been a

clandestine authoritarian turn, clandestine in a strange way, namely the chancellor saying for the first time,[4] that she is ready to go for hard measures and that she would do so on her own, without looking for any procedural legitimation. This comes up on different occasions during the interview, the first time it is mentioned, Merkel uses the words:

> *for me, this Monday with these consultations and the long breaks and many other things is also a caesura and it can't just go on like this: we meet every four weeks and continue in the same way and I think that's also the case for many minister presidents. ... but the implementation is not such that I am already convinced that this third wave will be broken and that's why the states have to step up. Otherwise I have to think about whether we can also find ways.* We have the infection protection law that we then specify again—**does that mean that you want to seize power?**—*I can't take power ... say the federal government must now have some kind of right of intervention ... no, that would mean constitutional amendments for which you can't get a majority at all. ... ... it always goes through the federal government and the states—either by means of mpk (conference of the ministers; P.H.) resolutions or by reconsidering whether we need to change something in a law and then have to pass it again in the Bundestag and the Bundesrat. That means it's always a collaboration between the federal government and the states; no one can take responsibility for it. But it all takes time and we don't have the time at the moment.*

(Merkel, Angela, 28.3.2021)

This raises serious concerns for two reasons. First and again, it is the question if and to which extent the so-called standards of Western democracy are compatible with the need to act effectively. Various slogans come to mind as 'democracy takes time'; 'if you want to go fast go alone, if you want to go far, go together'; or 'only measures carried by the will of the people, guarantee a smooth move forward'. However, it is easy to miss the point—later, the second argument, will underline this. Before coming to it, we should briefly point out the difficulty to define the demos, the will of the people, and the process of moving together.[5] In fact, we must look at the core issue of how any polity is constituted. Of course, this cannot be discussed in depth. The earlier remarks on the questionable 'constitutional process' of the new FRG may be called back to mind—not least because it is telling that the populist AFD is especially strong in those parts of Germany that are located in the region of the former GDR (while being to a large extent driven by 'invaders' from the former West).

---

[4] At least to the best of my knowledge for the first time.

[5] Mind the two possible meanings of moving together.

At least one further point should be raised, taken from debates on plebisc-itary and participatory democracy, referenda etc.. While there are surely good reasons speaking in favour of such concepts, there is in particular in today's soci-eties—highly complex agglomerations, confronted with the need to decide on multifarious issues—a dimension that has to be kept in mind.

maybe you are thinking that we live in completely different times today, where the citizen is not guided by emotions but by what is just and reasonable. Referenda would lead to the right results. I am afraid the reality is far from that. Social bots, i.e. small programs that pretend to be people, are independently on the move in the digital world; ... within seconds they can post thousands of comments and thus change the mood on the internet. ... most 18 to 29 year olds already prefer the so-called social media to inform themselves about daily events. In 2016, 57 percent of facebook users in Germany said that they mainly get information about politics from their facebook friends. And if I ask you now to imagine a man with a hat ......, you can't help it: you actually have a man with a hat in your mind now. Our world works like that because our brains work like that way: ... ; or think of our history: what to do when the democrats elect one (incomprehensibly), then such a decision is supposed to take precedence over a majority decision. ... ... when our consciousness developed, there was nothing to suggest that we would ever do anything different from our ancestors, the ape-men. If it had been according to the rules of nature, we would only have used our expanded abilities to continue killing the weaker ones, but we did something different—we set ourselves a goal. we created an ethic that does not favour the stronger, but protects the weaker. ... often enough we lose, again and again we fall back into the dull and animalistic ways of behaviour, but the magna charta, the declaration of civil rights, the bill of rights, these are our victories over ourselves. for them there was no model, nothing in nature indicated it and exactly this is what makes us human in the true, highest sense: the respect for our neighbouring human being. if today we are ready to give that up again because an absolute democracy seems easier to some, we are lost.

(von Schirach; translated P.H.)

One important point of reference in legal debates is the distinction between the categorical imperative and the consequential approach to decisions. Translating this into the question of the constitution of polities, communities, states and any form of 'social agglomeration', we should distinguish between an 'entity of decision making' and an 'entity orientating decisions'.

Ulrich Becker captures this multiple tensional field well, stating:

After all, times of crisis are not only times that require an effectively functioning state; they also require strong governments. It is true that political decision-making remains essential: restrictions on freedom must be legitimised just as much as the expansion of redistribution processes. In how far threats of the pandemic may be left to be handled by people on their own or require governmental intervention is not a simple fact but open for valuation and requires decisions, for which political responsibility must be assumed. It is also true that governments have to react effectively, and, in this sense, times of crises may also become times of strong administrations. Effectiveness is even a justification for policing measures and other restrictions of individual freedoms although the relation between those administrative actions and constitutional rights is not free from tensions. The same holds true for the relation between administrative and legislative powers. The urgency of security measures requires flexible and efficient action. As a consequence, statutory instruments and executive (delegated) legislation is gaining ground, sometimes to an extent which risks jeopardizing prior achievements in relation to the rule of law.

(Becker, Ulrich, November 2020 a: 11)

All this is not said to justify Merkel's course of action. However, we must turn our attention to the question of legitimation by procedure as it will be discussed more extensively below. Here it is only important to change the question. It is not about the justification of taking a single-handed decision; instead, the question must be concerned with the clarity of the process of authorisation.

Also, this is the second point, the lack of this clarity is a fertile ground for a fundamentalist critique that expands hopelessness, potentially completely paralysing policy making. Such position is brought forward by Giorgio Agamben, stating in the preface to small collection of texts under the title *A che punto siamo?* (Where are we standing now?).

More than four months after the start of the emergency, it is indeed time to consider the events we have witnessed in a broader historical perspective. If the powers that govern the world have decided to use the pretext of a pandemic - at this point, it does not matter whether real or simulated - to transform from top to bottom the paradigms of their government of men and things, it means that those models were in their eyes in progressive, inexorable decline and were no longer adequate to the new demands.

(Agamben, 2020 a; translation P.H.)

Later it will become clear that a generalist critique of government action as critique of authoritarianism leads paradoxically to authoritarianism, veiled in 'collective individualism/hedonism'.—Is it fair, then, to ask if we are facing a quandary? Speaking, as Agamben does, of a 'nuova religione della salute' (a new health religion); thinking of the victims, criticising policies of 'biosicurezza' (biosecurity) seems to be cynical.[6] However, it is an open question if and to which extent law can be used as reference and solution. The Kantian categorical

---

[6] Apparently he has some doubts too … would he otherwise write 'una pandemia—a questo punto non importa se vera o simulata—' ?

imperative had been presented as individualist and possibly amoral[7]; legal cases, confronting us with—cum grano salis—comparable dilemmas, are known from history. It is in particular the *case Queen v Dudley and Stephens (1884)* where we find the weighing up of lives and harsh measures of assessment and subsequent action. This case is completely different from Lon L. Fullers' widely known *Case of the Speluncean Explorers,* published in 1949 as a fictional case, presenting the moral dilemma of legal decisions *(see Fuller, 1949)*. Whereas in Fuller's fictional case the decision is about weighing up individual lives, applying the random principle to find a decision, the real case is about active choice against the will of concerned people, weighing up the 'qualified lives', suggesting the life of family fathers is more valuable than that of a young person who is most likely dying anyway.—Engaging more or less extensively in this issue is justified by two facts:

First, in future, with artificial intelligence playing increasingly a role, the general problematique of this case will play an important role and is similar to the moral dilemmas of politics and policy making in times of pandemics: we have—in order to programme AI—to decide ex ante about lives. In short: politics and policies that are not completely backed by the legal system, the triage as guiding the decisions of medical staff and decisions in digitalised settings will be part of daily life.

Linking this with the present discussion, we are dealing with the question if, to which extent and in which way the state has the right and obligation to intervene or at least to take action in the light of a threat to life; this question is made more complicated by the fact that in the case of pandemics it concerns • individual lives as such, • the lives of the members of society and • the live of individuals as determination of the lives of others. The German law constitutes on the one hand the duty of protection—this refers to the protection of the fundamental rights according to the Basic Law and—of limited interest here to para 241.2 civil code.[8] Of special relevance is the protection of life and physical (and psychological) integrity, secured by article *2.2 Basic Law ('Every person shall have the right to life and physical integrity. Freedom of the person shall be inviolable.')*. However, the same sentence contends *'These rights may be interfered with only pursuant to a law.'* This must be read in connection with article *1.1* and *1.2 Basic Law:*

---

[7] An easy, also for non-philosophers and non-jurists accessible presentation can be taken from *McEwan, 2019)*.

[8] The latter will be neglected—in the present context it would have some relevance insofar hospitals are subject to the control by the state while the relationship between the hospitals and the patients, the hospital staff and also the financiers as insurances is by and large a matter of private contracts.

(1) Human dignity shall be inviolable. To respect and protect it shall be the duty of all state authority.

(2) The German people therefore acknowledge inviolable and inalienable human rights as the basis of every community, of peace and of justice in the world.

The fundamental difficulty is given by the definition of dignity as brought forward by the Constitutional Court, emphasising the subject character of the individual and his/her independence which means, in turn, he/she cannot be made object of the state.[9]

First and foremost, this brings us back to the origins of human rights, emerging from the ambitious bourgeoisie, questioning the power of the feudal classes. In this light, HR are originally a defence of the bourgeoisie (then coalescing with the proletariat) against the feudal system—this is also manifested in the UDHR. However, it became more and more obvious that such conceptualisation misses the need to address the ongoing and varied processes of socialisation. Necessary is • a thorough consideration of the role of the state as key provider of certain services and as instance that secures—by active intervention—certain conditions; • that today enterprises are 'public actors' and as such also actors against the action of which human rights have to be defended, • to elaborate and emphasise the global perspective on human rights in a way that it is often not possible to name a 'single responsible instance'[10] and finally • a fundamentally new approach to understanding social rights (as part of the Human Rights agenda) as rights that go beyond (social) support of individuals.

In this light, the Triage-legislation is surely an important step. The Head-notes to the Order of the First Senate of the Federal Constitutional Court of 16 December 2021 highlight.

In the case at hand, the mandate of fundamental rights protection culminates in a specific duty to take protective action because there is a risk that persons will be disadvantaged on the basis of disability in the allocation of scarce, life-sustaining medical resources in intensive care.

3. Even when Article 3(3) second sentence of the Basic Law imposes a specific duty on the legislator to take protective action, the legislator enjoys a margin of assessment and appreciation as well as leeway to design, as long as it sufficiently ensures that

---

[9] Cf. BVerfGE [Constitutional Court] 115, 118—Luftsicherheitsgesetz; BVerfGE 30, 1—Abhörurteil; BVerfGE abw. M. [dissenting opinion] 30, 173; BVerfGE 50, 166; BVerfGE 109, 133—lebenslange Sicherheitsverwahrung.

[10] Though this should not be taken as excuse for an exculpation of individuals as it had been the case in an judgement concerning the Diesel-scandal *(see LTO-Redaktion, 27.06.2023).*

persons with disabilities are in fact protected against being disadvantaged on the basis of disability.

(Federal Constitutional Court, 2021)

However, we find a fundamental problematique the subsequent legislation does not address, with two dimensions:

- Practically it will be extremely difficult to implement this legislation as decisions have to be taken in most cases within an extremely limited timeframe, this limiting the possibility for consultation.
- Furthermore and structurally, the problem is that patients are—at least factually—too often classified as customers. Part of this is the notable role plaid by the pharmaceutical industry and more and more a pharmaceutical-technical complex *(see for instance Tansey, 9/2020; Jorgensen, 2013; Murray, 1974; Compton, 2023).*

The Corona State, Defining Itself

10

10.1 Some Economic Questions

10.1.1 Economy—Limits to the Analysis

Posing the question about a specific corona economy would have to look at two dimensions, namely a massive negative effect on the standard figures (GDP, employment, export …). To some extent the overall negative development had been temporarily cushioned by different factors that will be only viewed by highlighting some key factors.

* We can see a remarkable growth of online trade—and a relatively stable consumption especially until December 2020, probably strongly supported by the partial suspension of VAT-payments between the 1st of July and 30th of December 2020, as regulated in the stimulus package. Putting the VAT-suspension into a wider light, a qualification is needed, in particular in the perspective of fundamental rights. The website of the government states

> With the temporary reduction of VAT, the German government primarily wants to boost consumption again and give a new impetus to the German economy, which has been affected by the Corona pandemic. In addition to citizens, the reduction will also benefit businesses in all sectors, which will profit from additional purchases, from gastronomy to the automotive industry
>
> (Die Bundesregierung, 29.6.2020; translation P. H.)

According to the same source, the VAT accounts to approximately 1/3 of the total revenue. (1) How can it be justified, that an obviously huge amount of money can be mobilised to promote the economy while it had been supposedly scarcity

© The Author(s), under exclusive license to Springer Fachmedien Wiesbaden GmbH, part of Springer Nature 2023
P. Herrmann, *Pandemics as Matter of a System Crisis,* Prekarisierung und soziale Entkopplung – transdisziplinäre Studien,
https://doi.org/10.1007/978-3-658-43450-2_10

of resources that forced the privatisation of hospitals, introduced strict measures of rationalisation and resulted in the design of the health sector in a way that even the head of the Deutsche Städte- und Gemeindebund (German Federation of Cities and Communities) had to concede 'We are currently becoming more concerned about whether really economic efficiency is the decisive criterion, whether it is not necessary to say: We are going to maintain certain hospitals, even in the wider terrain.' *(Landsberg, March 11ᵗʰ, 2020; translation P. H.).* The development of the health sector is especially worrying as the privatisation puts the entire sector and not least the care staff under severe pressure, negatively effecting the rights of health care workers and patients alike: nurses in private hospitals earn 1,000 € less than the colleagues who are paid according to the tariff of the public services *(praktischArzt)—this is surely not because the payment in the public sector is extremely high;* the working conditions are in general hugely problematic as widely discussed *(see e.g. Quadbeck, 29.12.2020; with links to further documents)* (2) Reading that 'the reduction also benefits businesses in all sectors benefitting from additional purchases, from catering to the automotive industry' evokes the somewhat sardonic question how catering services are really benefitting the same way as car manufactures while they have to limit their business due to the lockdown, allowing them at most take-away business. As the IAB-study on *The impact of the Covid-19 pandemic: evidence from a new establishment survey* states

> the need to reduce personal contacts—at home as well as at the workplace—that has characterised the current crisis, also means that a wider range of sectors has been affected.
>
> *(IAB-Forum, 26.02.2021)*

This is clearly showing up in the development of the labour market—we learn from the same source

> A recent study has shown that regions with a larger share of employees in severely affected sectors, including accommodation and food services, experienced a larger increase in the net flows from employment into unemployment.
>
> *(IAB-Forum, 26.02.2021)*

Interestingly, the development of employment in the transportation and storage sector and ICT-sector had been negative. While this comes at first glance as a surprise, the explanation can be given by a closer look—evidencing the imbalances of the German economy in favour of large enterprises. For an understanding of this connection, we must look at the *so-called 'corona effect' ... defined as the difference in the annual change of the inflow rate from employment to unemployment and the outflow rate from unemployment into employment*

(Böhme, 2020: translation P. H.)

While at this stage any interpretation is limited by the fact that we are still looking at an ongoing process of which the long-term effects cannot yet be foreseen, the following seems to be likely: • losses seem to have occurred especially in the areas of small business service provision, not least due to the closure of many direct customer-related services (e.g. small restaurants and shops not asking for maintenance services); • independent of the pandemic, we find a process of centralisation that allows quasi-individualised applications being offered by big players; • the changed conditions for non-standard employment suggest that a shift of personnel to this end seems to be likely, entailing the danger of a structural long-term shift—such interpretation is backed by the development of patterns that are related to the gig-economy and also by the fact that we find in the transport sector an 'advance of the disenfranchised', often not even showing up in the labour market statistics (see also the reflections below on recognition of untypical work and new forms of employment). Many of these developments can also be seen as (temporary) peak of a more general restructuration of economic processes and structures, if not even as part of a formational shift, allowing the emergence of a new accumulation regime. Important is the understanding of and feeding into the complex totality underlying the current economic and also the behavioural and action patterns. We are witnessing the confrontation of forces, on the one hand pushing towards changes and on the other hand those striving for conservation and even retreat. At this stage, the winner of this struggle is by no means clear. The reason for this lack of clarity and predictability must be seen—amongst others—in the fact that any decisions taken at a moment can be justified by a specific societal rationale; however, as these rationales remain mostly somewhat clandestine, often not even known to the actors, who are often reduced on executors, viewers and/or character mask.

   * In fact, this leads to the next point: Instead of using the situation as opportunity for economic restructuring, implementing fundamental changes in order to gain sustainability, policies may be characterised as 'employment-first-strategy', maintaining employment especially by means of short-time work (applications

lodged in April 2020: 10.1 million, i.e. 26.9%).[1] The purpose of the short-time-work benefit was defined in the draft of the Employment Promotion Act (AFG)

> *The short-time allowance is granted to employees who suffer a loss of earnings due to a temporary loss of work in the enterprise caused by economic reasons or an unavoidable event. Its socio-political value lies in the fact that it reduces the insecurity of the employee's professional existence. In terms of economic policy, the short-time allowance, which preserves the labour force, serves to compensate for short-term economic fluctuations and to bridge structural changes in companies caused by economic developments. The significance of short-time allowance for labour market policy is that it stabilises employment relationships. On the other hand, short-time allowances must not disturb the natural selection process in the economy.*

> *(Deutscher Bundestag 5. Wahlperiode: 55)*

This means, that the current extension of the payment is in actual fact using the instrument without adequately reflecting the original goal laid down in the Social Code (SGB III. 6.1.1. §95 f.). The 'soft interpretation' suggests that this instrument was used for a policy, likely missing its economic goal: it turned out to be an instrument by which ailing businesses had been temporarily saved, often with little hope to sustain business in the long run. In other words: The core had not been saving employment but saving businesses. Thomas Sablowski highlights this aspect, saying:

> *The extension of the possibilities for short-time work was the first and most important measure taken by the federal government in favour of the capitalist class. This enables the capitalists to flexibly adjust their demand for labour to the dynamics of the crisis. They can suspend regular labour contracts and reduce their costs without laying off their wage-earning workers. They can reduce working hours at will and lay off some or all of their workers. Compared to laying off workers, short-time work has the advantage that when the situation returns to normal, capitalists can immediately fall back on their workers. This already proved its worth in the financial and economic crisis of 2008/ 09. By having the state pay short-time work benefits, the capitalists can pass on the payment of wages in part or in full to unemployment insurance or the state budget or taxpayers.*

> *(Sablowski: 524 f.; translation P. H.)*

---

[1] IAB-Forum, 16.4.2020—this document, and the links contained, offer much in depth information on the labour market development, including some references to the legal conditions.

A first glance at the statistics of insolvencies seems to back such an argument *(see Rudnicka/statista, 11.06.2021).* To some extent the labour market data point into the same direction.

The stricter interpretation suggests that we are witnessing a presumption of powers by using the instrument beyond the regulation defined in § 109 SGB III.

In addition, it must be seen that easy and unbureaucratic access had been granted in the framework of the stimulus package, however, the large share of various monies went to sectors of which the societal relevance may well be questioned—thus there is an obvious hiatus: in a general perspective we can welcome[2] the announcement of the promotion of a new green deal and learn about the intended use of the means from the EU-recovery fonds:

> *In justification, the EU Commission President said that the funding projects applied for by the German government would ensure that Germany emerges stronger from the corona crisis because it strengthens its future viability through digitisation and climate protection. In fact, the German government wants to invest more than half of the EU funds in digitisation.*
>
> *Chancellor Angela Merkel sees a need to catch up in administration, education and health care. Above all, the work of the health offices will be greatly changed by the EU funding, Merkel emphasised.*
>
> *(Ganslmeier/ARD, Stand: 22.06.2021 17:39 Uhr; translation P. H.)*

However, various factors should make us pay attention: why does all this stand under the aegis of maintaining German competitiveness? How can it be justified that air-traffic and car-manufacturing is heavily subsidised while the railway system suffers from underinvestment and discontinuation of some services and the rather efficient transport via canal navigation is still neglected? Can it be justified that private transport is still prioritised while radical approaches towards limiting private use of cars in the inner cities are at most limited to model projects? Comments on the digitisation strategy could be added, also highlighting shortcomings of policies that are geared to strengthening monopolistic competitiveness instead of a radical roll-out of citizen-oriented use of ICT and AI.

Taking together, we may have to face efficiency disadvantages: the reallocation of labour is reduced while unproductive companies remain on the market—short-time-work-benefit may well turn out to be state investment into ailing industries. This is especially remarkable against the background of the 'sale' of the former GDR-economy, the *Deutsche Treuhand* (trust agency, supervising the privatisation

---

[2] Though qualifications need to be discussed.

of the former state enterprises of the GDR), selling companies for one Mark—a
symbolic payment. Today—under the veil of the pandemics—we find the opposite: the state investing substantial money in industries and services that are
structurally ailing, the recent links only being an additional factor, accumulating
the negative factors.

• Born from necessity and expression of helplessness? This is, of course, an
  interpretation that is somewhat persuasive—who could deny that the outbreak
  of the Corona-crisis came abrupt and could in this form not have been predicted? Who could claim to have an ultimate program for maintaining the care
  of the population, while the situation had been characterised by increasing
  socio-economic demands and increasingly scarce—material and immaterial—
  means? Finally one had to deal with what was given and mistakes that had
  been made earlier acted now in a dictatorial way.—But as understandable
  such explanations are at first glance, a historical perspective opens the mind
  for another view. The spiritual-moral turn, introduced by the unholy trinity
  Reagan, Thatcher and Kohl in the late 1970s/early 1980s had been ultimately
  geared towards another goal than the supply of the citizens with necessary
  goods and services and the improvement of people's living conditions. Obviously, what Kohl put forward as idea of freedom, had been translated into a
  Wild West reality. The claim surely sounded at first glance reasonable:

> An economic order is all the more successful the more the state holds back and leaves
> the individual his freedom. The social market economy is better suited than any other
> order to realise equality of opportunity, property, prosperity and social progress. We
> do not want more state, but less; we do not want less, but more personal freedom.

> (Kohl, 1983: 57; translation P. H.)

The reality had been harsh and found in Germany an ultimate expression in
the work of the *Treuhand:* A gold rush atmosphere was systematically evoked,
characterising not only quasi-governmental policies but going much further, being
part and consequence of the move to the financialisation of the economy. It had
been not least a policy of easy money, going hand in hand with questionable
business practices by at least dubious figures and measures:

> Real estate agents posed as trustees, drove into companies and interrogated unsus-
> pecting employees about their real estate holdings. An alleged management consultant
> roamed the countryside, offering his services for 6,000 marks a day. The overtaxed
> East German clerks of a savings bank would in good faith grant any loan whenever a
> respectably dressed businessman with a business card promised to invest in the region.

> *Within a few weeks they paid out almost 700 million marks, among others 64 million to Stefan Stephan Grzimek, the son of the animal filmmaker, who wanted to buy 3 Boeing 737s to found an airline, that would operate from an airport near Hanover, which did not yet exist. A drinking hall operator from the Ruhr area received five million to open a window construction company in Halle.*
>
> *(Blasberg, 2022: 41; translation P. H.)*

But this had been just the exploitative abuse of a situation that stood on state-officially erected pillars: the number of privatisations as well as the speed of their implementation were remarkable. Later, even the overcoming of the division that had emerged in the course of this policy of taking over the former 'second German state'—the division • between East and West, • between those up there and those down there; • between those who were (some still and somehow, others as system rulers)—was to be done at the expense of those who had already lost at the beginning. 1997, Roman Herzog, at the time German president, suggested that

> *we need a new social contract for the benefit of the future. All, really all, vested interests must be put to the test. Everyone must move.*
>
> *(Herzog, 26.4.1997; translation P. H.)*

Becoming concrete, he asks for a society

> *in which the individual bears more responsibility for him-/herself and others, and in which s/he does not see this as burden but as opportunity?*

And he speaks of

> *a society of solidarity ...—not in the sense of maximising social transfers, but trusting in the responsible actions of each individual for himself and the community?*

It deserves mention that Herzog highlights that he sees time and location of his intervention indeed as matter of a new beginning.

* Social protection[3]: Looking at the numerous individual regulations would go beyond the scope of this contribution. Instead, the following will provide an outline of the main provisions, and in particular, at the structure of the measures, or one may say the politics of social corona-jurisdiction. At the very core, we

---

[3] This section owes much to the following two publications: Becker et altera/Max Planck Institute for Social Policy and Social Law, November 2020; ILO: COVID 19 ...;

find, as mentioned earlier, the orientation on maintaining employment or at least avoiding unemployment. The two pillars on which this orientation is based are (a) the easing of the introduction of short time work and (b) the lowering of the threshold and terms of conditionality. The draft of the bill in favour of easier access to social security and on the use and protection of social service providers due to the SARS-CoV-2 Coronavirus—'Social Protection Package'[4] states on page 2

> *Basic income support for jobseekers under Book II of the Social Code (SGB II) or subsistence assistance under Chapter III of Book XII of the Social Code (SGB XII) and basic income support in old age and in the event of reduced earning capacity under Chapter IV of SGB XII ensure subsistence if no priority assistance to cushion the economic effects due to COVID-19 is available. These benefits are to be made available quickly and in an unbureaucratic way in a simplified procedure in order to be able to support those affected promptly. No one should suffer existential hardship due to the economic effects of this crisis. The simplified procedure is necessary to support the job centres' ability to work. The simplified regulations should also apply to those entitled to social compensation. The adoption of the content of the transitional regulations of SGB II and SGB XII for supplementary assistance for subsistence in social compensation law under the Federal Victims' Pensions Act (BVG) ensures that comparable protection exists in all subsistence systems.*

This is later, on page 17, specified; we read

> *The economic impact can lead to people temporarily experiencing significant loss of income. This can affect all workers, but is particularly risky for the self-employed, and especially for small entrepreneurs and the so-called solo self-employed. This group of people usually has limited financial reserves and also has no access to other forms of protection such as unemployment, short-time work or insolvency benefits. As a result, an existentially threatening situation can arise in the short term.*

Looking at the measures taken in respect of employment and job security, we face an important contradiction: on the one hand we find an extension of relevant measures in particular when it comes to the need to take care of children—a need that is given by the closure of relevant services (creches, kindergardens, schools). According § 56 para. 1a IfSG, a person, taking care of the child and suffering from a loss of income, will receive a compensation of 67% of the average monthly income, though limited to a period of six weeks.[5] On the other hand, we find more

---

[4] Deutscher Bundestag Drucksache 19/18107 19. Wahlperiode.

[5] The time limit is the same 50 § 3 para. 1 Law on Continued Pay of Wages (Entgelt-fortzahlungsgesetz—EntgFG).

or less restrictive conditions when it comes to measures directed on the demand side of labour. While we may interpret the first set as more or less generous, we are witnessing on this side a restrictive approach, threatening further the position of workers.

These include, on the one hand, the expansion of marginal employment through the Social Protection Package, which is primarily intended to benefit the agricultural sector, the expansion of additional income opportunities for pensioners, the change in the crediting of income for recipients of student funds under the Federal Education Assistance Act (BAföG) and flexibilisation of parental leave. Another aspect is the increased flexibility of working hours basis of the COVID-19 Working Time Regulation, the working day can be extended, rest periods shortened and work on Sundays and public holidays can be arranged for. All this applies to certain activities which, in this context, are not labelled as 'system-relevant' but are listed in detail as being in the special general interest

(Becker, November 2020: 29 f.)[6]

* An important aspect, while being difficult to grasp, had been of major interest, concerning the perception of 'relevance for the system'. It is difficult to determine what is relevant for the system—philosophically one may even distinguish between relevant for the system itself and relevant for people living in the system. Pragmatically, food supply and medical services are obviously relevant; the classification of books as especially relevant as means of social communication *(see Lederer, Klaus, 3.3.2021: minute 6 ff.)* and the subsequent exceptional opening of bookshops in Berlin *(see Pressemitteilung vom 14.12.2020;* https://www.berlin.de/rbmskzl/aktuelles/pressemitteilungen/2020/pressemitteilung.1030169.php; *12/07/2021)* are an example, showing the possible width as it is easy to move on from here to cinemas, theatres, public readings .... Hairdressing may be considered being part of personal hygiene, what is then with care of nails? If not seeing this as matter of hygiene in the strict sense, one may easily argue that it is an issue for mental hygiene. Presenting these examples is intentionally provocative, showing that there are two layers, politics has to consider: the first is to define what cannot be defined, i.e. to provide clear definitions and clearly present used criteria; the second is to apply them on the executive level. This goes far beyond allowing hairdressers to open, and nail studies not; it becomes interesting especially

---

[6] The threshold for additional earnings had been also raised for 2021; qualifying: Die Anhebung der Hinzuverdienstgrenzen gilt für Neu- und Bestandsrentnerinnen und -rentner. Keine Änderungen gibt es hingegen bei den Hinzuverdienstregelungen für Renten wegen verminderter Erwerbsfähigkeit und bei der Anrechnung von Einkommen auf Hinterbliebenenrenten.—see Deutsche Rentenversicherung, 12.01.2021.

while debating (human) rights, when we include the wider area of industries. Is maintaining the production of cars system relevant, exposing workers to the various risks? Indeed, here system relevance may be only defined as the car industry being relevant for the system: a sector standing at the core of the economy—from here one comes immediately to the question if maintaining *this* economy is more important than the security rights of the workers.

Then, again on a pragmatic level, we must see the question of 'fair renumeration'. Many of the positions at the core of system relevant areas (medical service providers, grocery store shop assistants, transport workers …) are especially exposed to infection; but they proved to be underfunded and in many cases even precarious. Precarity especially in this field deserves attention, as many of the transport workers, increasingly important due to the mentioned boost in online-trade, are working under conditions that are in various ways highly problematic (undercutting minimum wages, occupational safety and health, working hours, social security …). On the positive side some changes must be mentioned:

- An increase of the income of care and cleaning staff in hospitals remains an unanswered demand. However, we find at least a Corona bonus in 2020 and also 2021. Instead of rewarding directly the employees, the money is paid to hospitals, these then being responsible for the distribution to their employees, reflecting their exposure to special risk and requirements.
- Recognition of untypical work and new forms of employment is another topic—some progress can be seen as some previously unprotected forms of employment are now 'de-precaritised', and included in the various security systems.

It is remarkable to which extent the entire situation depends on definitions. A study by the IAB suggests that in Germany non-standard forms of employment are a marginal issue and do not play a role, then, however, speaking of temporary contracts:

> The share of fix-term contracts fell significantly between 2018 and 2020 as a 2021 study by Christian Hohendanner shows. Short-term employment contracts with a duration of less than three months are hardly relevant in Germany.
>
> (Bruckmeier/d'Andria/Konle-Seidl, 28.05.2021: 2)

On the other hand, they emphasise the increase of

new work arrangements such as on-call work or casual work, mobile work using information and communication technologies (ICT) or freelance work under work contracts or service contracts. These new forms of work, mainly ICT-based mobile work, have grown exponentially during the Covid-19 pandemic and associated lockdown measures, although they are not a new phenomenon.

(Bruckmeier/d'Andria/Konle-Seidl, 28.05.2021: 3)

It is equally important to consider the context—for instance, the high percentage of part-time work as well as the fact that long-term unemployment had been already since some time high, thus massive lay-offs could be avoided.

For the time being it is fair to say that teleworking as a more or less new field confronts us as well with several uncertainties. The OECD reveals in its *Employment Outlook 2021* the following figures (Fig. 10.1 and Fig. 10.2):

Currently the problem is that these figures must be adjusted with two other figures—at the moment this has to remain limited as the figures specifically for Germany are not available.

Furthermore, the following must be considered: a huge number of previously employed people has moved out of the labour market—which may mean that

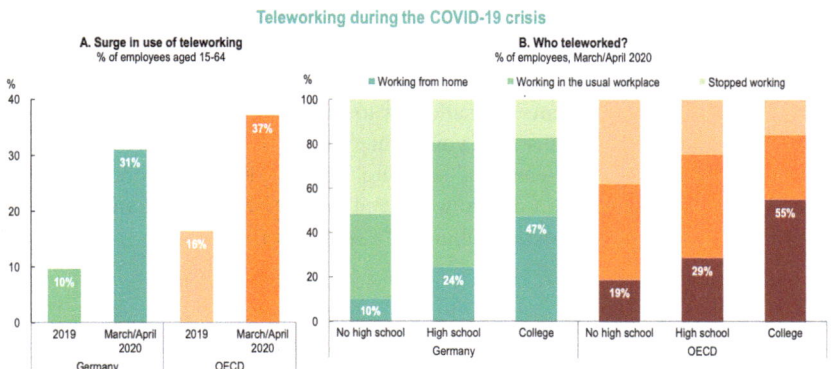

(Scarpetta/Carcillo, 08.07.2021: slide 9)

Fig. 10.1 Massive Use of Telework, but not for all *(Scarpetta/Carcillo, 08.07.2021: slide 9)*

The impact has been uneven, heavily affecting youth and the low-paid (low-educated)

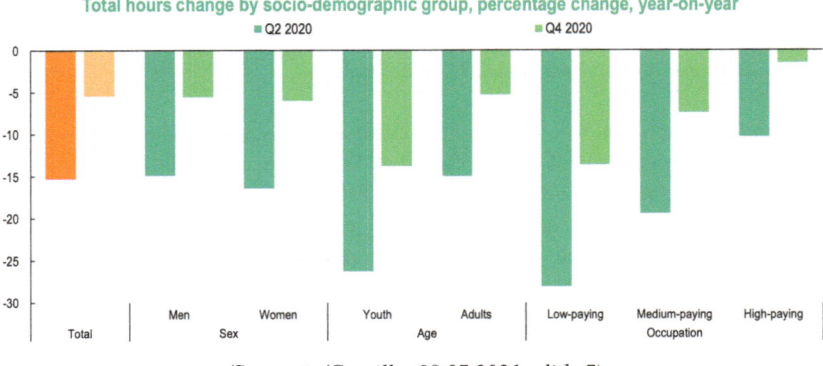

(Scarpetta/Carcillo, 08.07.2021: slide 7)

Fig. 10.2 Impact of Telework *(Scarpetta/Carcillo, 08.07.2021: slide 7)*

they really moved entirely out of employment or it may mean that they are now in positions that do not show up in the statistics.[7]

At the end, though, there is time for a cynical remark: what is the reason behind giving pensioner's opportunities for additional income? In a good willing interpretation, we may say that the standard security, given by the pension system, is not sufficient and they are now allowed to increase a low pension; however, we may also say—and this is the cynical interpretation—that old age pensioners are now sacrificed in the name of securing the execution of work for which nobody else is available. This can go well hand in hand with the argument brought forward in a different context, speaking of a societal triage.[8]

10.1.2   A Spiritual-Economic Turn?

What follows is more a reflection coming from an anecdotal and impressionist perspective—it can be doubted if anything more systematic is possible at all: (α) certain reactions had been just this: reactions in the sense of adapting behaviour

---

[7] In this context also of interest: ILO, 2020.

[8] See Herrmann, 2021.

to given circumstances, without changing fundamentally the attitudes; (β) conditions changed in a very short period, thus not giving sufficient time for certain trends to develop towards a sustainable structural change; (γ) conditions, modes of processing and reactions had been locally/regionally very different but also different in respect of social strata, thus making any real empirical analysis questionable; (δ) some phenomena being part of general and secular trends, making us however more sensitive to perceiving and even overestimating them, while we are not sufficiently able or willing to link questions of power, structural moves of economic and professional development, secular and generational changes and systematically integrate the contradictions, including forces and contradictions of 2nd and 3rd order.

Looking at the recent economic development, we may speak in some respect of a kind of spiritual turn or even multiple spiritual turns. Using such wording requires a warning: we have to be aware of the continuity throughout the entire period, linking all discussions back to pre-Covid 19 setting the standard for what is normal, while there had been at the same time considerations of a new development, a new stage of economic structuration of capitalism or even its end, at least its end as global system, in other words: a system in need of regionalisation.[9] We find hand in hand with these debates considerations regarding the role of the state. After the unquestioned and seemingly unquestionable dominance of the (mostly so-called) neoliberal ideology with its specific monopolist-globalist role of the state we find an increasing tendency to revisit this role: social equalisation and compensation payments[10] are put again on the agenda, as the means for individual self-sufficiency from earned income is obviously reaching its limits, now also including strata that used to be considered to be reasonably well-off; at the same time, however, economic subsidies are increasingly considered, specifically geared to small and medium-sized enterprises; in connection with this, orientations towards local and regional suppliers are articulated, in turn being accompanied by special quality issues (quality of production, working conditions and products). This moved even to considerations regarding the validity and meaning of standard success measurements, in particular GDP, on the agenda.

---

[9] This latter factor has in Germany a special meaning as it is interwoven with the takeover of the former socialist country by the FRG—part of this had been for instance the denouncing of the quality of products from the Eastern Laender, Western supermarket chains opening shops in the former GDR, now 'importing' milk from the Western Laender.

[10] Going beyond those transfers that are 'normal' in a state in which social (including health) insurance and tax financed payments play a major role.

Another ongoing topic had been the question of system relevance: which jobs, which economic activities are really relevant for society and for the economy, relevant and needed to secure the functioning of society.

We must look at these questions in connection with a general or secular trend, namely the increasingly pressing environmental challenges, and in the meantime also the consequences of the war between Russia and Ukraine, challenges we all face globally. To some extent this had been linked directly with issues around the pandemics: Alluding to and borrowing from Ulrich Beck it may be said that a virus is as democratic as pollution, both being characterised by not knowing any borders. And the danger of an escalating war is by no means completely off-beat as Western forces are already since a long time and completely independent from the current manifest confrontation showing a perceived need for geopolitical clarification, playing down hegemonic claims *(in this context Solty, 1.3.2023: 12, arguing against a half-heartedly-lied, ahistorical assessment of the situation and Ukraine).*

10.1.2.1 Excursus: The Tragedy of the Media—Their Abuse as Means of Mediating Sedation—The Larger Tragedy is the Cal(a)m(ity) of Communication

Although these are central aspects of the overall development in objective terms— and concerning the objective conditions, another aspect is given by changing the stage of the various 'performances'. Already this formulation provides a hint— we are talking about politics and policies as matter of performances, looking for stages that allow public-pleasing appearance. Commenting on the *Talk Show Sabine Christiansen,*[11] we read in the article *Sabines Welt,* written by Klaus Boldt and Wolfgang Hirn *(Boldt/Hirn, 31.10.2003, 18.00 h)*

> *Bundestag President Wolfgang Thierse therefore refers to 'Christiansen' only as a 'substitute parliament' and warns of the addictive dangers of TV appearances as only a man with a full beard can warn. He calls talk shows 'importance drugs'.*

Noteworthy is that the broadcaster ARD assigned the talk-show to the resort entertainment, not politics; the broadcast is produced by an independent producer, thus not immediately and fully under control of the public broadcaster. *Mais-chberger* (previously *maischberger. die woche* and *Menschen bei Maischberger)* is not direct successor but in fact successor of a talk-show that was explicitly meant to be entertainment *(Alfred Bioleks Boulevard Bio).* Bottom line is that it

---

[11] A political talk show, broadcasted at prime time from January 1998 until June 2007.

is another 'staged polit-show'—staged and staging, as it is today standard: the idea is that the show must go on, and it will only go on if politics and policies are presented in the format of entertainment, lightening the serious character (i.e. responsibility) and the threatening consequences of politics and policy-making, while establishing a kind of re-medialisation, or at least re-feudalisation.

- Cum grano salis, the same applies for Anne Will's show, where Merkel had been regular guest, in a position to ask for being invited, and using it as platform suitable to announce that democratic rules do not necessarily have to be respected. It had been mentioned earlier that she said that in case of doubt she would revise jointly made decisions and subordinate them to her view.

Going beyond this tragedy of the media—their abuse as means of mediating sedation—the larger tragedy is the cal(a)m(ity) of communication. Traditionally, the German polity had been characterised by at least claiming the maintenance of a system of mass media as 'fourth estate', complementing legislative, judicative and executive power. The idea behind it had been expressed by the Basic Law and its interpretation by the Constitutional Court. In its judgement from 1958 the court states.

> As the most direct expression of the human personality in society, the fundamental right to freedom of expression is one of the most noble human rights of all (un des droits les plus précieux de l 'homme according to Article 11 of the Declaration of the Rights of Man and of the Citizen of 1789). It is the very essence of a liberal-democratic state order, because it makes possible the constant intellectual debate, the battle of opinions, which is its lifeblood (BVerfGE 5, 85 [205]). In a certain sense, it is the basis of all freedom, 'the matrix, the indispensable condition of nearly every other form of freedom' (Cardozo).
>
> (BVerfG, Beschluss des Ersten Senats vom 15. Januar 1958; translation P. H.)

The headnotes of the judgement emphasise that

> Fundamental rights are primarily defensive rights of the individual against the state. However, the fundamental rights of the Basic Law are also an expression of an objective order of constitutional values that amounts to a fundamental constitutional decision and therefore applies to all areas of law.
>
> (Abstract of the Federal Constitutional Court's Judgement of 15 January 1958)

The same court, specifies for the

> *The responsible participation of citizens in the political decision-making process of the*
> *nation presupposes that the individual knows enough about the issues to be decided,*
> *about the decisions, measures and proposals for solutions made by the established*
> *state organs, to be able to judge, approve or reject them. Public relations work by*
> *the state can also make an essential contribution to this. The more the individual is*
> *thus called upon to make his or her own judgement, and the more he or she is made*
> *aware that, as a responsible member of the legal community, he or she can influence*
> *the shaping, formulation and concretisation of the legal order that is binding for all,*
> *and that he or she can participate in fundamental political decisions, the easier it will*
> *be for him or her to accept as his or her own the state established by the Basic Law,*
> *which offers him or her these possibilities.*
>
> *(BVerfG, 1977; translation P. H.)*

In consequence, the media governed by public law (öffentlich-rechtliche Medienanstalten) had been—and still are—obliged to balance the provision of governmental information, general publicity and neutrality/objectivity.

However, this claim had been, in fact at least, borne to the grave. Instead, the public media are now watering information on politics, policies and policy making down to entertainment and decisively translating it into a binary scheme: the good and the bad, the real and the irreal ..., all based on the presumption of interpreting decisions in the light of unavoidable technical matters.

Commenting on the talk show Sabine Christiansen, Susanne Gaschke fears in the weekly newspaper *Die Zeit* the antipolitical resentment as keynote and states, also quoting the moderator.

> *She, the media woman, likes to make herself the advocate of the imagined citizens*
> *living the country. The indecisiveness of many voters is the result of an 'over-staging*
> *of politics', says Christiansen, 'if we already experience show-like performances in*
> *the Bundesrat, in the political institutions, we don't have to be surprised if there are*
> *similar attempts in the media. Indeed, but: does a more artificial event, one more*
> *dependent on staging, exist than a television talk show?*
>
> *(Gaschke, Aktualisiert am 29. November 2013, 21:21 Uhr; translation P. H.)*

And Burkhard Spinnen, writing in Die Welt, sees the

> *weekly public liquidation of what was once political discourse.*
>
> *(Spinnen, 22.06.2007; translation P. H.)*

He concludes

Sabine Christiansen was the moderator of the futile attempts of functionaries to still speak politically as they once did under the reign of constraint. She was the chaperone of a company outing of full-time desperate people. While she was liquidating the political conversation in a forced, serious and nonchalant manner, she was at the same time consoling over this execution. Her conclusion was not that in the end the curtain falls and all questions (unfortunately!) remain open; her message was rather that one can settle into failure as long as it is moderated with decency.

(Spinnen, 22.06.2007; translation P. H.)

This suffocation of the public discourse reflects the breathlessness of the supposed function of the parliament, namely the function as controlling entity of the government: The resources for parliamentarians (academics working for elected representatives …) are insufficient, the expertise comes from the executive and lobbyists so that independent work of parliamentarians is at least difficult, more a private pleasure of the individual representatives. Political questions had been redefined, baptised as TINA, suggesting that there is no alternative, which had been true in the shadow of the following basic consensus: (a) Germany has to be competitive in economic terms, i.e. under the premiss that

[t]he wealth of those societies in which the capitalist mode of production prevails, presents itself as 'an immense accumulation of commodities,'[.] its unit being a single commodity.

(Marx, 1867: 45)

(b) that the international reputation and reliability in the eyes of other countries is more important than the will of the people—expressed by Angela Merkel in the words (talking about the immensely contested railway station project in Stuttgart:

If this project would not be realised, we would no longer be considered reliable. If I, as Federal Chancellor, then say at the European level: 'Because there was so much protest here, unfortunately we can no longer keep what we promised', then tomorrow my Greek colleague will come and say: 'Because there was so much protest here, I can no longer keep the stability culture'. I certainly don't want to risk that.

(Merkel, 28. 9. 2010; translation P. H.)

The citizen—in the parliamentarian system and media representation alike—is increasingly seen as disruptive factor, a nuisance,

. treated as a negligible quantity, or merely as an entry in a statistical table or on a balance sheet, which is to say mute objects about which political decisions are made.

(Eribon, 2013: 132)

As stated earlier: the show must go on, and it does so by presenting politics and policies in the format of entertainment, lightening the serious character (i.e. responsibility) and the threatening consequences of politics and policy-making, while establishing a kind of re-medialisation, or at least re-feudalisation. The good and the bad, the truth and the lie ... binary, non-discursive 'factual issues', demanding forms of digitisation and supporting their introduction and suggesting directly or indirectly that political decisions can be reduced on algorithmic computations—a variation and continuation of what is widely discussed under terms as post-truth politics, post-reality politics and post-factual politics.

10.1.3   Phasing—More Than a Chronology

With respect to the pandemics, we can distinguish between at least six different phases.

10.1.3.1   Initial Phase

We may speak of a first initial phase, commencing with people becoming—after a phase of relative denial—aware of the danger caused by the virus itself and equally by the challenge to manage it. Especially when politicians got aware of the threat and talked publicly about it, we saw a kind of shock, fear and helplessness. While this had been first and foremost a matter of dealing with the situation, feeling confronted with questions of every day's life—supply with groceries, a somewhat strange obsession of hoarding toilet paper,[12] doing physical exercises, walking the dog etc.—there had been on another level the 'difficulty to accept the pandemic as pandemic'[13] *(Liessmann, 25.1.2021; translation P. H.).* As Konrad Paul Liessmann states:

> *It also affects the self-image of our society. In this self-image, such an event as this pandemic was actually no longer foreseen. It actually contradicts our concept of security, of health, of advanced medicine and medical technology. It also contradicts our expectations of the community, of the state, that health care will work and can be*

---

[12] It is mentioned here as it may be worthwhile in another context to reflect on a possible connection between the authoritarian character (see Adorno et altera, 1950) and what may be 'hygiene as obsession'.

[13] German original: Tun uns schwer, die Pandemie als Pandemie zu begreifen.

guaranteed. Illness has been an individual problem in these advanced societies, but it has not been a social or even a political problem.

One aspect of this grievance, this feeling of being offended, this feeling of being unpleasantly touched, this feeling of being angry about all what the pandemic is doing to us and has brought upon us, is this mistrust now of medicine, of science, of the promises of progress and safety in which we had actually settled very well and very comfortably.

(Ibid.)

10.1.3.2 Initial Phase 2

The initial phase 2 is quite different: we find the ongoing shock, but now it is complemented by notions of benevolence—benevolence by ordinary people and also benevolence as topic raised by politicians, issuing a strategy resting on three pillars: • the call for solidarity,[14] • the plea for rational behaviour, where rationality had been backed by reference to the Robert-Koch-Institute and its research by virologists and • the threat and execution of restrictive policies. The rational backing had been not really thought through in a strategic manner when it comes to legal and especially economic aspects. Looking at the reactions of the population,[15] we find different notions of solidarity: collaboration, co-funding of initiatives, support of local shops etc., surely based on different motivations. These reached from changing perceptions, i.e. recognising poverty on the streets which had overlooked previously, fear of sliding into a situation where oneself needs help, pure, especially Christian, benevolence ('a good life here will be rewarded there') and surely as well a kind of condescension behind the notion of the better-off strata, stating this way that 'We can do it'.[16] It can be said that in all these cases a strong sense of rejecting moving on in the 'rails of the old normal' functioned as underlying attitude. This went hand in hand with the growing awareness of the long-term character of the pandemics and even the fear of entering a 'pandemic era'.

10.1.3.3 Accommodation

A third phase can be seen as phase of accommodation, getting along with the new situation for which obviously a simple solution within a short period of time

---

[14] Mind: not practicing solidarity.

[15] Which is of course problematic because we find very different strata.

[16] Replicating on the individual level Merkel's statement from the declaration on the occasion of the role of the migration policy (see Merkel, 2015).

would not be available and of which the course and the 'final solution' cannot even be predicted today. Is it cynical, humorous or ridiculing to say 'people felt secure, after being assured that there would be enough toilet paper for everybody'? Still, this accommodation phase included in the early phase uncertainty about the *post-covid normal* and how this would relate to the *pre-covid 19 normal*. – Indeed—as briefly touched upon earlier –, there is some notion of a turning point in time.

Despite the general imponderability, many people felt more or less secure. In terms of income, we find mixed feelings and knowledge about support provided by state agencies; relatively little came from voluntary or welfare associations as they had been struggling as well, due to the shortcuts of social protection systems and increased needs. Various issues need to be considered in this respect; few will be mentioned (see already the earlier presentation).

- Reduced working hours had been the most common reply, strongly supported by enterprises and relevant government bodies. Surely, this meant for many a relief, and even rights-based security. Taking a wider view on the economy, however, it may be questioned if this had been a wise policy, if in actual fact the right to obtain a secure place in society, including a reasonably secure perspective, is undermined. The problem is that we are challenged to think about the concrete understanding of rights: in the present case we may speak of a tension between rights of individuals to short-term security, the rights of individuals to obtain a perspective, the right and obligation of society to guarantee security and the right and obligation to develop a safe place. In any case, this is also hugely relevant for determining the character of the state and the definition of dignity—a topic dealt with on another occasion in the present work.
- The handling of some grants occurred to be problematic—or should one say that some grants proved problematic? Anecdotal evidence shows that money had been distributed in an unbureaucratic way, also without delay but we could see as well that it had been impossible to benefit from relevant schemes as there had been so many applicants that only a small number could be served— seen in a wider perspective one may say that administrative and procedural requirements and laws require a careful coordination with issues of justice in a wider sense.
- Home office—at least for some time for many a 'new normal'—involves several issues. Questions around insurance had to be solved; more fundamental:

the home must be defined as workplace which may in extreme cases contradict substantially the right to a private sphere. This is a matter of defining physical space but also of time. Equally relevant is the question of taxation of space and reimbursement for office material, use of the private phone, additional cost for nutrition in cases where there is would be otherwise a canteen and the assessment of the time needed to go to the copy shop, post office and the like. By and large some rules do exist regarding taxation: under restrictive conditions a separate room or 'distinct space' can be claimed in the tax return for deductions.[17] But before it comes to this question, another question is relevant: using space for commercial purpose is subject to the landlords' agreement.[18] This will not be further discussed while at least two aspects must be highlighted as especially important: 1) there are blurring borders and it requires additional energy, usually from the employee, to find a way through

---

[17] Principal restriction on tax deductions for home offices: (§ 4 Abs. 5 Nr. 6b EStG in Verbindung mit § 9 Abs. 5 EStG).
Exceptions as tax allowable expenses:
* If no other workplace is available for your professional or business activities, you can claim your costs up to 1250 euros per year (limited deduction).
* If the office space is the centre of your entire professional or business activity, your costs are deductible without limitation.
(Reuss, 16.4.2021; translation: P. H.).
Revison, 9.12.2020 (Corona-Pauschale fuer home office beschlossen Finanzen/ Ausschuss—10.12.2020; 1370/2020 https://www.bundestag.de/presse/hib/812718-812718; 01/07/21).

'If the taxpayer's home office does not meet the requirements for the deduction of expenses for a home office, the taxpayer may deduct a flat-rate amount of five euros for each calendar day on which he or she performs all of his or her business or professional activities exclusively in the home office.'
With the home office lump sum as part of the employee lump sum, an unbureaucratic tax consideration of home work is made possible for the years 2020 and 2021. The Corona pandemic forces a great many people to pursue their business or professional activities at home. The new regulation provides for a flat-rate deduction of 5 euros/day, a maximum of 600 euros per year—which corresponds to 120 home-working days—as business expenses or income-related expenses. The lump sum is only granted for the days on which work was exclusively done at home. Travel expenses (e.g. commuting allowance) are generally not deductible for these days; expenses for an annual ticket for public transport, if purchased in anticipation of its use for commuting to work, are deductible regardless. The home office lump sum is also offset against the income-related expenses lump sum.
(Bundesministerium für Finanzen Jahressteuergesetz 2020).
[18] Qualifying: BGH, Urteil v. 14.7.2009, Az. VIII ZR 165/08.

the jungle of administrative and other rules; 2) the relationship between private and non-private sphere is blurred. Importantly this is not only a question of relevance for the employee and his/her relationship to employer and state respectively. In addition, we can easily see a loophole, employers availing of subventions without using this term. We may get a glimpse of the dimension of such shift when we learn

> *The Commission very quickly saw the potential benefits of perpetuating this situation. Without any social dialogue, without any real consultation, and even without any full information, and above all without any evaluation of the impact of telework, neither on the real quality of the work done under such conditions, nor on the physical and psychological health of the staff, the Commission decided to introduce profound changes in working methods.*

> *These changes include: a reduced physical presence, open-plan offices, the generalisation of 'dynamic' offices—i.e. hot desking –, the elimination of most canteens, collective spaces in general, and even the eventual reduction of central crèches or day-care centres...*

> *The aim is clear: to reduce the number of occupied buildings from over 50 in 2020 to 25 in 2030. In terms of the number of square metres, this would mean a reduction from some 780,000 square metres to less than 580,000. In financial terms, the savings would be around €440 million.*

> *(Union pour l'Unité, 25/05/2021; translation P. H.)*

In short: *'the Commission will slash its portfolio by 50% by 2030'* (see in this context: *Office re-entry is proving trickier than last year's abrupt exit; in: The Economist; 28/06/2021;* https://www.economist.com/business/2021/06/28/office-re-entry-is-prov...cloud&utm_term=2021-06-28&utm_content=article-link-1& etear=nl_today_1; *29/06/2021).*

We may even say that home-office entails the danger that the formerly private ownership of the accommodation will now be dissolved—based on tax and insurance law; a kind of cold expropriation without referring final responsibility to the new owner.

• Issues arise around communication—the legally relevant aspects can be summarised by highlighting the following keywords, only mentioning some of the problems: * surveillance, * increasing pressure—the extension of working time and difficulty to 'keep distance from one's self' (traditionally discussed as issue of work-life-balance), * substantially orienting on 'streamlining', making assessment easier, which means in turn—most likely—cutting-off qualitative and complex part of the work, their externalisation and with this most likely an eternalisation of 2nd order, for instance public services being (in part) outsourced, the service provider—actually being only an intermediary—stripping complex issues down, so that they can be easily handled, ideally automated with use of digital technology so that the user/customer has to put things together, provide information in a computerised format. We all know the often-endless menu-based information requests when calling administrations, institutions, businesses—legally it means that we move from an 'obligation to provide' *('Bringschuld')* to 'provision that has to be sought' *('Holschuld')*. This relation, common in contract law, is now applied in the area of public service provision, thus fundamentally changing the relationship between state and citizen, but also between employer and employee. Leaving the detailed meaning aside, we are confronted with at least two fundamental issues—they have to be mentioned although it is unlikely that an indisputable answer can be found: the first is dignity, resulting from the changing function and role of the state and its position as employer; the other is the concern with personality rights and the lack of their recognition by a system of externalisation of two orders, resulting in a tension between empowerment on the one hand and disrespect of personal concerns.

- While there are many more threats of the said kind, another dimension of accommodation can be seen in the increasing awareness of the potential dangers and the quest for regulations that aim on a clear and rights-based regulation, probably the most virulent is the quest for the right to disconnect—now not a matter of academic discussions but increasingly—and in its complexity—recognised as matter urgently to be resolved. The right to disconnect is not only seen as matter of the overall working time but also as issue of Occupational Safety and Health (OSH).

- The initial insecurity and psychological distress turned for many at some stage to the redefinition of priorities of life. While on the one hand—for instance by the OECD, (not least social-democratic) think-tanks and academics—the question 'Der Arbeitsmarkt nach Corona—was braucht es für einen tragfähigen Aufschwung?' (The post-corona labour market: What is needed for a viable recovery?) *(e.g. OECD Berlin Centre and Institute for Employment Research—Research Institute of the Federal Employment Agency: 08/07/2021)* had been raised, another notion had been the ventilation of issues beyond employment. One point worthwhile to be mentioned is a resurge of DIY-activities. Interestingly enough, building-supply centres had been without major restrictions accessible throughout the entire time—equally relevant: professional work and activities of private households apparently represent a special value and a specifically high reputation. Also, the choice of holiday destinations changed, much supported by advertisement campaigns. Special mention deserves that holidays 'near to home' had been strongly campaigned for, not least by the Deutsche Bahn, the successor of the national state railway company, without being backed by especially attractive prices. Also, this stands in stark contrast to the massive financial support to the main national air carrier, namely Lufthansa.—Still, we may face some value shift. On the other hand, the reaction may also be the opposite, tempting to travel in the future 'now more than ever'.

10.1.3.4 First Relief

The next phase has been perceived by many as relief—lifting of the lockdown, the possibility to return to shops, though with some remaining restrictions and in many cases one main restriction, namely long queues. It seemed to be like the first shot of a drug addict after some time of forced abstinence, underlining how deep-seated consumerism is, and also showing that consumption is here and now much more than purchasing, in fact being an important form of socialisation. It is surely worthwhile to mention and investigate more in detail the underlying soci(et)al stratification of patterns of consumerism. This would allow not least to investigate more in detail some questions of participation and empowerment. Is it fair to say that consumption is an attempted way to compensate for lacking other rights of participation? Or in a stronger formulation: as far as we can go with T. H. Marshall's suggestion of rights, developing from civil to political to social rights *(see Marshall, 1950),* we can see an inversion: with a factual restriction of civil and political rights, insisting on social rights is becoming more important, even if it is only a faked form of social rights, namely the 'right to spend money'. In this context, 'factual restriction of civil and political rights' may be a matter of direct restriction, the explicit prohibition of freedom of speech or equally relevant: the factual exclusion as consequence of uncontrollable complexities (bureaucratic requirements, juridification …) (see in this context for instance McDonald/Cranor: 2008

10.1.3.5 Re-Accommodation

By and large, later a new lockdown had been again accepted and answered in a disciplined way and we come to another period of re-accommodation, people becoming more aware of the fact of a long-term issue, affecting the entire life—in this way we may speak of some notion of potential new normal: living in a less consumption-oriented economy or at least taking different routes of consumption, also trying to rationalise this by way of referring to environmental needs, while also becoming more 'modest', appreciating time for the family, doing things in the house/accommodation (for those who have) etc.. And it had been definitely the period of the emerging online trade boom; especially those who have been already strong in the online sales became even stronger; nevertheless, other businesses moved also online, not as serious competitor of the main players but reflecting that online trade had been definitely not only the future but showing up already as presence. Having highlighted the general patience, we have to see also an increasing awareness of contradictions—or an increasing factuality of contradictions and the reason for them, namely a lack of strategic thinking combined with mismanagement: why is it possible for hairdressers to have their shops open but not for beauty salons? what is or what can be done about schooling, about kindergardens, how can we accommodate this with day-to-day's challenges and tasks of parents? .... There had been many of these contradictions and difficulties, causing impatience. Even if it had been by and large not a broad political movement, it became more prevalent that people looked for some niches, loopholes or ways of getting along with as little interruption as possible: what can we do to have at least individual satisfaction in the situation and how can we deal with it? There was another brief period of opening and a new lockdown—for some time it seemed to be fair to see in the middle of 2021 the last phase being reached, preparing to return to the pre-Covid 19 stage. It meant as well that that less considerations about different ways of life had been raised. From the outset of that phase it was safe to say that online shopping will remain high even if the opening of shops and especially of areas where social meetings are taking place means a huge relief. Finally, shopping is not primarily about buying goods: with the production of exchange taking the unquestioned priority before use value, socialisation and exhibition is taking over as primary goal of shopping.[19] Still, we find also some considerations as well in respect of traveling: 'we don't have to go for large, long-distance trips, making holidays in foreign countries—we can enjoy holidays just around the corner.' All this is well reflected throughout the entire time in advertisements.—It would or will be interesting, having at some stage a detailed study of the development of this sector, first emphasising solidarity, mutual responsibility and as well societal responsibility, celebrating the heroes of every day's life, but then returning to the 'old normal'.

  An objectified approach had been taken by *The Economist,* offering a *Global Normalcy Index,* explicitly defining the pre-pandemic level

---

[19] A statement one can make without buying into the thesis of *The Society of Singularities (Reckwitz).*

as 100 *(see* https://www.economist.com/graphic-detail/tracking-the-return-to-nor malcy-after-covid-19; *13/07/2021).* Still, one may also see it as cynical, as it disregards all previous notions of critical assessments of the old normal, accepting several of the shortfalls that the crisis management brought with it (e.g. the shift towards online trade and the subsequent pressure on SMEs and increasing negative environmental consequences; or the airline traffic still low, thus lowering the overall 'performance').

10.1.3.6 Settlement in Uncertainty and Precarity

It is difficult to highlight a specific time, defining a turning point. One may speak of a process of gradual habituation—not primarily regarding the virus itself (though this is also relevant, even in the second half of 2023) but primarily to the lack of security and predictability. It is probably fair to say that governmental politics and policies resulted in an attitude of toleration: While representatives of the system walked literally over dead bodies, they claimed that this would be the only and ultimate possibility to save the economy as the foundation of societal production and reproduction. Importantly, this was by no means a matter of adhering to so-called neoliberal policy patterns. Rather, they were quickly prepared to throw the basic principles of this orientation overboard—replacing them by an explicitly pro-monopolistic strategy, without a social and societal veil. In other words, economic growth in a national(ist) perspective had been presented as ultimate goal, putting the actual interest in securing supply first. Important is the fact that in this perspective the economic interest had been more than ever highlighted, denying the 'social dimension' and difference when it comes to specifying the interest in supply.

Alexander Dibelius, a medical doctor, later then heading the German office of Goldman Sachs, asked in his new role, representing the private-equity fonds CVC if it is justified.

> that ten per cent of the—really threatened—population are spared, but 90 per cent together with the entire national economy are extremely hindered, with the possibly dramatic consequence that the basis of our general prosperity is massively and permanently eroded?
>
> (Dibelius, 27.3.2020; translation, P. H.)

Of special interest is the link, Dibelius establishes between—capitalist—economy and human rights, suggesting

> *For centuries, we have fought at all levels for our individual freedom, for laws and human rights. And suddenly much of this is wiped away virtually overnight. How and when are we supposed to weigh these individual goods against each other: optimal health protection of a subgroup, general promise of prosperity and individual freedom rights?*

(Dibelius, 27.3.2020; translation, P. H.)

Indeed, we may feel reminded of what Adam Smith wrote in his opus magnum about the then new order:

> *… commerce and manufactures gradually introduced order and good government, and with them the liberty and security of individuals, among the inhabitants of the country, who had before lived almost in a continual state of war with their neighbours, and of servile dependency upon their superiors. This, though it has been the least observed, is by far the most important of all their effects.*

(Smith, 1776: 412)

Instead of neoliberalism, at least in the meantime a more or less useless 'concept' due to its undifferentiated overuse *(see for a critical analysis Birch, 2017),* we witness a new renaissance, now not looking back to ancient times but referring to the anxiety driven and anxiety enhancing times of early capitalism. It is also interesting that at a time where a virus spreads globally, breaking down all borders, nationalists and nationalism come to new glory.

10.1.4   Economics—not Even Changing the Wineskins

At this stage it will be clear, that the question of change—its scale, scope and action—cannot be clearly answered. For many, at least for a relevant group of commentators from academia, general public, mass media and also politics, it is clear that the so-called neoliberalist strategy and its suggested mindset, in some respect officially launched by Helmut Kohl's demand for an intellectual and moral turning point,[20] reached its limits. A recent study, going beyond the crisis linked to the pandemics, suggests that

---

[20] During the election campaign 1980 Helmut Kohl asked for a geistig-moralische Wende (intellectual and moral turning point). While the concrete meaning remained open, the principal orientation had been marked by • turning away from the welfare state, • calls for responsible citizens, suggesting that—as individual—every man is the architect of his own fortune [and here the conservative ideology argued actually in a gender-neutral way, applying this rule also for the fate of women] and • maintaining state intervention, though orienting it

> *[e]mpirical evidence indicates that significant parts of these crises are linked to the downsides **of the long-held market-liberal paradigm** that guided policymaking across most of the world for at least three decades. As with comparable moments of transition from the past and knowing that societies rely on an overall leitmotif[.] to function in trust, this collapse of a paradigm has left a dangerous vacuum—a **paradigmatic vacuum** that **populists** are trying to fill using simplistic answers without really addressing the challenges generated by this failure.*
>
> *(Fricke, et altera, 2023: 1; emphasis in the original)*

However, reading the report itself means facing diverse moral and normative hopes, rational conclusions and demands … but ignores by and large the power question and the fact of vested interests as main factor, determining what is seen as rational. By and large, so the argument here, the entire notion underlying the outline of an *Emerging Socio-Economic Paradigm Shift* remains within the framework of traditional economic approaches, erected on supporting pillars as scarcity, markets being determined by balancing supply and demand, rational economic (economically rational) actors, to be more precise: the homo economicus, separation of exchange value from use value, in tendency equalising macro- and microeconomic praxis, referring to the state as last resort. While some qualifications do apply, these are supporting pillars and too often only few parameters are changed, to be more precise: slightly altered. Marked evidence is the frequent reference made to the war economy.

Corona economics—it is in fact questionable to suggest that something like it, i.e. a turn of economic thinking, really exists. In many respects it seems to be even a more conservative trend; germs of alternatives, today frequently termed heterodox thinking, had been faster victims of fighting corona than fighting the virus. Remarkable are nevertheless the following trends, though emerging since some time, but becoming more meaningful now—only some keywords will be mentioned:

* The debate on 'heterodox' and 'green economics' got in some ways mainstreamed, though this had been more a consequence of a slow learning progress, emerging from the mid-2000-crisis, than a matter of sudden wisdom. The underlying problem may be summarised by the following: finance industry does as such not produce any relevant values; this was getting even more obvious as inequality increased, with poverty mushrooming and not least—due to tax policies—the question of the 1960s/1970s re-emerged, namely the question of public debt and private wealth *(see for the early debates O'Connor, 1973; also Streeck July 2013).*

(under the veil of growth, international competitiveness and suggesting trickle-down effects) on measures favourable for major export-oriented conglomerations.

Part of this constellation had been that redistribution reached such scale and shape that the triple movement—• financialisation of everything (including for instance health), • open and clandestine subvention of selected industries (including the exploitation of state-financed basic research, public infrastructure) and • the massive pressure and fiscal requirements coming from general[21] challenges (in particular environment-related matters), but as well the new dimensions of the means and modes of production especially given by new technologies as digitisation and artificial intelligence and with the dominance of online-business, moving the 'real economy' even further away—meant that without revisiting fundamental questions, even mentioning sustainability would be a waste of time.

* Behavioural economists gained in recent decades a stronger position in economics, after Herbert Simon (1978) and Gary Becker (1992), celebrating the first breakthrough probably with Daniel Kahneman and Amos Tversky in 2002, followed by Richard Thaler in 2017.[22] This links to the previous point: it became increasingly obvious that economic analysis cannot be limited on a narrow take on the relationship of rational individuals in the marketplace as locus of balancing demand and supply.

* A further qualification of the market-society emerged from the experience that global chains are fragile: obviously the high degree of dependence caused major problems for the globally connected German economy (depending on imports from the periphery and oriented on exports on the world market). In short, the pandemics put questions of regionalisation, localisation and different forms of growth on the agenda—many arguments that could potentially also be used in favour of protectionism. Indeed, as much as we are talking about the fragility of the Western benefits, we have to see as well the pressure emerging from the global system, namely the capitalist success story of so-called threshold countries.

* Re-valuation of work and exploring 'relevance for the system', meaning its function in a narrow sense, had been another issue—though mainly discussed as matter of actual policies, and not even from heterodox sides with a serious notion of restructuring of the fundamentals of renumeration of paid work. An exception, though not playing a major role, can be seen in the debate on UBI.

Taking all these factors together, highlights the need to theorise the relationship between public and private in the economy, thus being of course of immediate relevance for jurisprudence and answers to possible future challenges

---

[21] General as in global and affecting all strata, areas of societal existence …

[22] Robert J. Schiller (2013), also behavioural economist, had been left out as his work is geared to a rather specific field.

as we witnessed with the pandemics. The question of centralism or federalism will then be more like industrialism versus financialism.

10.2   Lost lives—lost living?

We find far-reaching critical positions from the earliest time of the virus' occurrence and reaching from a fundamental denial to the critique of individual measures, experienced inconsistencies and not least expressing only some personal impatience.

Far reaching denial had been already mentioned earlier, with reference to Giorgio Agamben. It is probably justified to distinguish between four lines of critique:

- The well-founded worries about side-effects and counter-intuitive collateral damage, often going hand in hand with personal insecurity about handling personal situations. One example is the difficulty of living under extremely restrictive conditions and the need to look after the child/the children who would normally be at least for some time be looked after in a crèche, kindergarden or school, now also being deprived of their social contacts and support of homework
- A radicalisation of such questioning, simply denying the danger of the virus and emphasising the negative effects of the control of the pandemics
- A politicisation of the critique, not dealing with virological/medical aspects but with a specific direction of political measures, namely their restrictive character of which it had been said that they are restricting fundamental rights of individual self-determination, and thus the disrespect of personal freedom as highest value of a dignified life
- The radicalised politisation, suggesting that the virus would be used as excuse for a coup d'état—an argument brought forward by forces of the extreme (new) right

There are no clear demarcation lines between the four types of critique; realistically we are dealing with a scale that is for two reasons of special relevance.

(α) part of the critique is in one or another way justified—'in one or another way' may look like the following, taking up on the example mentioned earlier, namely the conditions of accommodation. Obviously, such constellation is problematic. However, it is equally problematic to see this as purely virus-related matter. Instead, it is more correct to issue this as problem of housing and school policies. The justification is even more given when people make the experience that those problems do not find any place where they can be addressed, that for instance the municipal offices, dealing with housing issues, are not accessible or that rent seeking speculation is unhindered on the rise.—At least a temporary reaction can be seen in the following:

> *late or oustanding payments of lessees between April 1st 2020 and June 30th 2020 may not result in a termination of the rental agreement for 24 month. However debts must be paid until June 30th 2022 or cancellations may take place.*
>
> *(ILO: COVID 19 and the world of work. Country Policy Responses)*

Long-term, we see the introduction of the legal entitlement to all-day services for primary school children as of 2026: while this had been already pursued since 2017, the debate and the process of decision making had been accelerated (https://www.bundesregierung.de/breg-en/search/all-day-care-at-primary-schools-to-be-expanded-1911210; *13/07/2021; Gesetz zur Errichtung des Sondervermögens 'Ausbau ganztägiger Bildungs- und Betreuungsangebote für Kinder im Grundschulalter' (Ganztagsfinanzierungsgesetz—GaFG), BGBl, Nr. 61 vom 14. Dezember 2020;).*

(β) Part of the critique is not and does not relate to the pandemics—it is a more fundamental critique of modernity in its current form. One dimension is the critique of culture—blurring the borders between the here and now and secular processes. The other—here of special relevance—is about the limits of the legal system. In the same spirit as Anatole France speaks of *[l]a majestueuse égalité des lois, qui interdit au riche comme au pauvre de coucher sous les ponts, de mendier dans les rues et de voler du pain (France, 1894),* we can speak of the de-substantialisation of the constitutional state, subject to the formalisation and juridification. Taking Montesquieu's formula of the separation of power as point of reference, we arrive soon at the problem that is similar to the one we know from the socio-economic analysis presented by Károly Polányi. In a nutshell, he emphasises—and critically questions—a market, solely geared to and steered by monetary gain:

> *The true criticism of market society is not that it was based on economics — in a sense, every and any society must be based on it — but that its economy was based on self-interest. Such an organization of economic life is entirely unnatural, in the strictly empirical sense of exceptional.*

...

Actually, as we now know, the behavior of man both in his primitive state and right through the course of history has been almost the opposite from that implied in this view. Frank H. Knight's 'no specifically human motive is economic' applies not only to social life in general, but even to economic life itself.

(Polanyi, 1944: 249 f.)

This market society is cut-off any societal and social control, though the latter is in some way reintroduced by way of welfare provisions *(see ibid.; cf. Fraser, 2012; Fraser, 2013)*. We can reformulate this, saying that the entire economy shifted from (re-)producing daily life to (re-)producing the distributive circle, separating the production for use from the production for gain, while back-staging the first.[23] Cum grano salis, the same is happening with a polity that is characterised by the separation of powers: While (and even if) legislature, executive and judiciary are well balanced, i.e. controlling each other, they are limited to what Niklas Luhmann called legitimation by procedure. In this light, law appears as problematic when it comes to the search for solutions of democracy and equally of substantial issues as that of a global health threat. The real problem may be clandestine, hidden by the veil we are wearing as supposed protection. To get an understanding of 'legitimation by procedure', we can refer to Luhmann's presentation of *Law as Social System*.

The repeated use of communicated meaning fulfils a double requirement: the results are, finally, a meaning that is affixed by language and differentiated societal communication. On the one hand, such repeated uses of meaning must condense the used description in order to make sure that the meaning is recognised as the same, even in a different context. This leads to the surplus of references, which can be shown in the direct experience, and which render any concrete fixed definition of meaning impossible; all future use of the references, then, comes under the pressure to be selected for such use.[.] In a highly abstract form, this is a description of the genesis of meaning.[.] Only those who participate in this logic of condensation and confirmation of meaning can participate in communication by language and can thus couple their consciousness with social operations.

(Luhmann, 1993: 144)

---

[23] If we refer to Marx' *Grundrisse*, we may say, that production in the wider understanding is segregated into its four elements and reduced on consumption, redistribution and exchange, leaving production outside of the consideration.

And later this finds its expression in the brief formula that 'the function of law produces a binary scheme in which normative expectations, whatever their origin, are fulfilled or disappointed … ' *(ibid.: 174)*. What Polanyi says about the market society, is with view on the legal system already expressed by Cicero in his *De Legibus,* saying.

> *Quintus:—You take up precisely from above and, as is fitting, brother, from the same source, what we ask; and those who teach civil law differently, teach not so much the ways of justice as the ways of quarrelling. Mark: Not so, Quintus; it is ignorance of the law rather than knowledge of it that is the source of quarrels. But this will be discussed later; now let us look at the foundations of law. It pleased the men who were still learned in the matter to start from the law, I do not know if with good reason, provided that, according to their own definition, the law consists of the supreme norm inherent in nature, which orders what is to be done and forbids the contrary. This very norm, when it is made certain and impressed on the human mind, is the law.*

(translation, P. H.)

Because law is today welded into a binary code, only committed to a legal discourse, it may be assumed that this hopelessness is the real reason behind the judgement by the Federal Constitutional Court on the problematique of triage. Triage, in general terms, may be understood as the spontaneous, even instinctive, decision by medical staff, confronted with the choice of helping one or another person, limited by the available capacities. Of course, even then there are certain criteria applied, though they may reach from affect, i.e. personal sympathy over physical ease to reach relevant equipment needed for an intervention to sober estimation of the 'effect' any choice has to help, i.e. help the patient to survive (being afterwards able to lead a dignified life). If time allows, the answer to the question will of course not be given by an individual but by a group or team, being in a position to decide rationally. The question the Constitutional Court had to answer, had been about the need for an explicit[24] regulation of the triage by law. The problematique is obvious: • the legislator, i.e. the state, would decide about dignity, with this interfere with the inviolability of the personality *(see the earlier discussion of articles 1.1. and 1.2. of the Basic Law)*[25]; • the criteria that are necessarily part of such legislation, would automatically entail a definition of dignity and thus criteria by which different individual lives are weighed—this could

---

[24] Explicitly, meaning going beyond the general legislation that is regulating (para-)medical professions.

[25] Detailed discussion would need to consider also the legislation of professional obligations and limits defined for instance in connection with patient's provision.

be the likelihood of saving a life, the number of years saved by an intervention, the 'net worth' of a person, the social meaning/relevance for instance measured by family members (children, elderly …) the person cares for and the like; • such general definition of criteria would be problematic in terms of equality but also in terms of de-contextualisation, quasi-objectivation and de-situationalisation of a decision.

(γ) Fear of total surveillance is another critical aspect—critical in the understanding of an area where critical voices are raised but also critical assessments are easily missing the point.

A recent survey, undertaken by the *IfD Allensbach—Institut fuer Demoskopie* –, the leading German pollster organisation with a quasi-official status, found a major decline of the share of the population that sees the fundamental right of freedom of opinion granted *(Petersen, IdA, updated 16.06.2021–05:53).* While there is an obvious link between the decline and the pandemics, it should not be overlooked that (i) it is part of a more general trend and (ii) that during this period divergent opinions on a topic, that is of immediate relevance for everybody, came to the fore, thus making by its very nature disputes and their limitation more visible[26] and also directly requiring everybody to take a position (even not necessarily publicly). Such climate provides a fertile soil for polemical remarks as those made by Giorgio Agamben, suggesting:

> *I am certainly not alone in thinking that, for a totalitarian government like China's, the epidemic was the ideal tool to test the possibility of isolating and controlling an entire region. And that in Europe we can refer to China as a model to follow only shows the degree of political irresponsibility into which fear has thrown us. And one should question the rather strange fact that the Chinese government declares the epidemic closed when it sees fit.*
>
> *(Agamben, 2020 b; translation P. H.)*

The challenging part of this constellation is that especially those who criticise(d) the surveillance, complain(ed) also about the lack of public control (i.e. control of the public in its appearance of [mostly] statutory bodies) and the limitation of freedom of opinion where such freedom is seen in close connection or even as part of a right to privacy and at the very same time as means of control

---

[26] Furthermore, other highly controversial topics (e.g. racism, migration, CO2-emmission, data protection) plaid an equally important role, pointing into the same direction.

of the public. In addition, referring another time to Agamben,[27] he frequently highlights the importance of the separation of power as ultimate mechanism of control of political processes, stating that 'il principio della divisione dei poteri su cui si fonda la democrazia.' *(Nuove riflessioni*[28] *"Neue Zürcher Zeitung", 27 aprile 2020).*

On this ground, we may reformulate the question of protection of privacy and freedom of opinion. In a simple formulation we can suggest that we are dealing with a deconstruction of privacy and the obligation of opinion. As this will be easily misunderstood, the following short explanation will be given: while there are surely areas that are private in the sense of not (necessarily) be talked about with others, at least not with any other person, the ontological point of departure must be that humans are social beings, and that means that some kind of public is given by definition. The proposal is that, instead of artificially separating humans from the public, we must accept publicity and design it in a socially responsible way. In other words, the task is not to escape from the public, but to consciously design it, together with others, also accepting controversial disputes. In turn, this means the obligation to formulate opinions, arguments and being ready to their defence. Information matters, of course; while not following Pierre Bourdieu's 'concept de capital' *(see Bourdieu, 2000),* it is surely important to emphasise that capital can control information and education but information and education can also control capital at least to some extent. Control mechanisms in this respect

---

[27] The reason for this reference is given by the fact that he seems to be a widely acknowledged chief ideologue of Corona-critical voices across Europe, without any doubt bringing forward some 'thought-through arguments' whereas his German contemporary, Gunnar Kaiser, is surely qualified for making noise but not in developing sound arguments. Another point to be mentioned, but not more than in a footnote: some attempts had been made to establish a new party, e.g. Widerstand 2020, WiR 2020—so-called Querdenker are gaining some ground. The reason for not engaging is simple: leaving aside that the apparently new phenomenon has a history in the 'Wutbuerger', defined as 'expression of a sceptical centre, that aims on maintaining what they have and know' Ausdruck einer skeptischen Mitte, die bewahren will, was sie hat und kennt, [Kurbjuweit, 2010: 26 f; also: Stimmenfang #163], resulting not least from the tranquilising politics by Merkel, answered by conspiracy theories; leaving also aside if these parties may have any long-term meaning, and leaving also aside if they may develop at some stage beyond an institution that is focused on only one programmatic issue, they are here seen as not primarily Corona-related but part of a far-reaching shift in the political landscape, the analysis of which goes beyond this contribution although it may well be seen to be part of the narrative used here, namely the disclosure of hidden—historical and contemporary—mechanisms of a structurally precarious polity resulting in the breaking trust.

[28] L'articolo riprende e svolge il testo di un'intervista pubblicata sul quotidiano "La Verità" il 21 aprile 2020.

are surely important. But at present the interest is directed to the forgoing stage, namely the need to acknowledge that information beyond the formal process is necessary. While this presupposes the separation of state and citizen—as condition of the establishment of dignity in the understanding of the Constitutional Court—this distinction is, in turn, condition for the usefulness of the legal system. Ernst Wolfgang Böckenförde elaborated this as separation of the state as political instance from the citizens, who, in consequence of this separation, are able to define themselves as free individuals *(Böckenförde, 1967; also: 1973)*. In a provocative interpretation we can speak of the withering away of the people, the state establishing itself as quasi-independent power. Of course, this formulation contradicts fundamentally Böckenförde's intention. On the contrary, the free individual is the critical force which the state cannot create, however being crucially in need of it. But to the extent to which the state becomes independent and is reduced on a formal instrument for the execution of power, another need emerges: the withering away of the state as separate instance and the (re)integration of its functions into society—Evgeny Pashukanis reflected the contradictory process extensively *(see Pashukanis, 1924)*.

10.3   Economy and Society

Max Weber's seminal work, titled *Economy and Society,* may be taken as point of reference. However, here it is not about an interpretative approach to society, but an interpretative notion towards managing life under the conditions of pandemics. The era of enjoying a retreat of ten days[29] is gone—or if re-feudalisation is a reality, it did not return yet (entirely[30]). Obviously—and this became clear at an early stage—we are not looking at a period of a very limited time; equally clear is the fact that such retreat is impossible in a world with a highly differentiated economic system.

In addition to the briefly mentioned online trade, in some ways as complement, we find some forms of new 'niche-ism': the search and creation of niches. We can speak at least of two phenomena that are important enough to classify them as trends.

---

[29] Alluding to Giovanni Boccaccio's Decameron.

[30] Such statement is safe, even if Branson, to be precise Sir Richard Branson, escapes on private mission for a 1.5 h space flight (https://www.bbc.com/news/science-environment-577 90040; 13/07/2021).

The one is the search for, 'falling into' niches that are best described as the offer of the 'crumbs that fall from their masters table' *(Matthew 15.27):* these are in many cases precarious positions and options as free rider. Indeed, it is often about delivery jobs, legally as contractors, this way allowing the main haulers saving on taxes, social contributions etc.. The responsibility for substandard working conditions, breaching laws that are dealing with Occupational Safety and Health (OSH), minimum standards when it comes to working conditions, income and social insurance *(see for instance Paketfahrer ...; Flüchtlinge als Paketzusteller ...; TV Doku ...; Doku—Undercover ...; Lieferdienste ...; the documentations refer to different dates, clearly evidencing that the phenomenon is not new, though it is likely that the situation is more problematic now).*

The other is the search for 'real niches'—one example is a small start-up in Berlin, offering • services especially for older people with no or limited affinity to computer, internet use and smart phones, thus especially disadvantaged under the condition of an increasing relevance of IT/ICT, • reading groups, talking about books, chosen by the participants and • an 'Erzaehlcafé', an online meeting, open to everybody, aiming on exchange on a variety of topics, in some way one may say a version of the Philosophische Stammtisch, broadcasted by the SRF1 *(Schweizer Radio und Fernsehen; Swiss Radio and TV Broadcasting* https://www.srf.ch/play/tv/sendung/sternstunde-philosophie?id= b7705a5d-4b68-4cb1-9404-03932cd8d569*; 27/06/2021),* bringing experts of their personal life (also known as wo/men in the street) together for a participative exchange of experiences, views and knowledges). Some of the work is financed as paid service, part voluntary activity, to some extent financed through private donations from participants *(see for this example the website of the enterprise and a report in a leading German weekly journal:* www.silber-salon.de[31]*; Plitz, 2021).*

---

[31] The self-presentation reads: Der Silber Salon ist eine Plattform für digitale Bildung und ein generationsübergreifendes Netzwerk, das 2020 während des Lockdowns gegründet wurde. Unsere Mission ist es, gemäß den 17 Zielen der Vereinten Nationen, insbesondere 3 (Wohlergehen), 4 (Bildung) und 10 (Chancengleichheit), der älteren Generation den Zugang zur Online-Welt zu ermöglichen, um digitale Chancengleichheit zu schaffen.

Wir helfen der älteren Generation mit einer großen Portion Humor, in leichter Sprache und mit viel Geduld, Teil des digitalen Zeitalters zu werden und bauen zugleich Brücken zwischen Jung und Alt. (https://www.silber-salon.de/%C3%BCber; 27.06.21).

Finale

It is surely not that; though it may well be that we are witnessing a kind of Grande Slam. Indeed, it is a highly competitive tournament: • human nature against an aggressive tumour; • human nature searching for a balanced sustainable lifestyle that accepts the power of nature and the limited ability to control it; the contest for equality, allowing to take care of resources in a way that limits the spread of such decease and secures to the largest extent possible the health and security of all citizens, globally. All this is not least a matter of human rights and their new conceptualisation. Such new conceptualisation, first, needs to accept that talking of universal human rights was and is increasingly problematic, as we can learn from Karl Marx, arguing in the first volume of *The Capital* against Proudhon:

> *Proudhon begins by taking his ideal of Justice, of 'justice éternelle', from the juridical relations that correspond to the production of commodities: thereby, it may be noted, he proves, to the consolation of all good citizens, that the production of commodities is a form of production as everlasting as justice. Then he turns round and seeks to reform the actual production of commodities, and the actual legal system corresponding thereto, in accordance with this ideal. ... Do we really know any more about 'usury', when we say it contradicts 'justice éternelle', 'équité éternelle', 'mutualité éternelle', and other 'vérités éternelles' than the fathers of the church did when they said it was incompatible with 'grâce éternelle', 'foi éternelle', and 'la volonté éternelle de Dieu'?*

(Marx, 1867: 96)

Second, with this in mind we must look at the fact that human rights are about a social and class struggle, taking the form of a 'struggle for law' and a struggle

P. Herrmann, *Pandemics as Matter of a System Crisis,* Prekarisierung und soziale Entkopplung – transdisziplinäre Studien, https://doi.org/10.1007/978-3-658-43450-2_11

between different dimensions of justice, in particular the individualist and the social(ist) perspective.

Third, while it may well be contested that human rights can be elaborated as universal rights, there cannot be any doubt that any debate must be globally oriented.

Fourth, while the forgoing analysis is far from being complete, looking at all the detailed regulations, it will definitely be clear at this stage that such debate is (a) about daily life, (b) has to go beyond a strictly juridical perspective and (c) has to take not least a historical perspective.

Fifth, precarity can now be seen as part of a new normal. Saying so, we should not overlook that it is not so new. More correct is to speak of a change of forms. In a nutshell it is the permanent activation of the reserve army of the working class—where working class must be taken in a wide sense, reaching across all groups of people being economically dependent. Hand in hand with this restructuration goes a paradox movement: while for—real and potential— wage earners risk is privatised, i.e. everybody is to the highest degree obliged to look for and accept ways that allow generating some income, the—real or potential—employers are discharged: the many and increasing cases of so-called working poor can be taken as indication.

It is surprising then that even from the left critique and proposals fundamentally following the traditional line of capitalism, and only suggesting that growth is the necessary and even only solution to current problems. For instance, Thomas Sablowski highlights the economic crisis, especially concerned with the lack of growth: the assessment is based on the analysis of the standard parameters, especially the GDP. He states at the end of that contribution the limitation of such approach, suggesting the need for a more fundamental change:

> *Finally, it is important to point out once again that the distortions of the current crisis are largely not caused by the Corona pandemic as such, but by the fact that it is taking place in societies dominated by the capitalist mode of production.(.) Any society that stops parts of its production for a few months in order to contain a pandemic thereby loses part of its material wealth. But it makes a big difference whether an 'association of free people', 'working with communal means of production and self-confidently spending their many individual labour forces as one social labour force', decides in solidarity what is really important, what restrictions on production and labour are necessary and possible, which areas of social reproduction must be maintained at all costs, and how the problems that arise can be overcome together, or whether the individual and private enterprises in capitalist competition ultimately remain on their own, while the state takes emergency compensatory action and distributes the available resources according to the social power relations.*

(Sablowski, op.cit.: 539; with reference to Marx, 1890: 92)

However, even here there is no clear recognition of the *Critique of the Political Economy* – this is the subtitle of *Marx' Capital*. The first volume begins by highlighting the fact that the wealth of capitalist nations is showing itself by the immense accumulation of commodities

In the same book he contends later:

> *If we presuppose communal production, the time factor naturally remains essential. The less time society requires to produce corn, livestock, etc., the more time it wins for other production, material or spiritual. As with a single individual, the comprehensiveness of its development, its pleasures and its activities depends upon the saving of time. Ultimately, all economy is a matter of economy of time.*

(Marx, 1857-61: 109)

Indeed, seeing the political economy of the pandemics in connection with Human Rights is highly important: instead of assessing economic progress only as matter of accumulation of commodities, we must direct the attention to gaining time: securing individuals' lives, securing lives of historical subjects that control production and reproduction of daily life instead of being controlled by the capitalist order and its executives where the focus is given by the production of commodities and the reproduction of the economic circle. Precarity can now be redefined—and the Covid-crisis did not change anything, it only highlighted issues, this is the summarising thesis: it marked for a long time society, not primarily as matter of labour market related issue but as structural problem of the polity: an institutional system that is by and large incapable to act. In this light, precarious working and living conditions are indeed only of a secondary character. It remains true that we are dealing with the consequences of economic development and insufficient reflection in policy making; but decisively the precarity of the political system itself provides the framework and consequence, marking everything by the same structure, leading to the feeling of subjection and discontent ... and opening the political stage for right-wing, populist movements and doctrines. Thus, the challenge is not to find measures geared to integrate those who became disintegrated, but indeed the major challenge is the need to overcome the disintegration of society. The guideline along which this can be discussed is given by the social quality approach and it's for objective factors namely socio-economic security, cohesion, inclusion and empowerment. Keeping this in mind, the following are fundamental tensional lines, along which societal integrity must be considered—as such they provide a framework for developing further the discussion about human rights.

First, societal integrity is about establishing a framework of security which includes the protection of the relevant public. While this requires an autonomous institutional system, able to act independently, it goes hand in hand with the requirement of being a protected system in the sense of being protected against the influence of vested interests.

Second, we are facing the need of a structurating system, which itself is structured (i) by law and (ii) the process of structuration itself—one may think of the re-solution between status and contract, life world and system world and communicative acts. However, it will be necessary to develop these discussions further instead of looking for simple ways of application.

Third, one fact for the need of revisiting the concept of nation state—as socio-economic, political, and legal entity—is the process of globalisation. It is currently limited by institutional frameworks that are—once acting is liberators—turning into fetters of further liberation. Approached with caution, debates on governance can be helpful.

Fourth, this is accompanied by the tension between totality and particularity, again and again discussed as question of diversity as matter of necessary respect of the other standing against the need of uniforming forces as condition for cohesion.

Fifth, we must look at the productive tension between social and individual forces. While the mainstream in social science refers in this respect to methodological individualism, and an initial answer may consist in the reference to mythological socialism, further consideration will lead us again to the importance of recognising the social as

> outcome of the interaction between people (constituted as actors) and their constructed and natural environment. Its subject matter refers to people's interrelated productive and reproductive relationships. In other words, the constitutive interdependency between processes of self- realisation and processes governing the formation of collective identities is a condition for the social and its progress or decline.
>
> (van der Maesen; Walker, 2012: 260)

Important is to approach these tensional lines in a relational way—seeing them as horizontally and vertically mutually reinforcing and controlling. In a relational perspective we are not talking about contradictions but the opening for productive processuality.

If we return to the reference to a grande slam, there is surely one major obstacle when using such metaphor: here can only be one winner, and that is mankind; anything below that would be the 'Waterloo of humanity'.

In the Prussian state, the dynasty has politically based itself on the status of the Prussian Junker right up to the present day.

(From the Inaugural Lecture Max Weber's, 1859 in Freiburg; translation, P.H.)

Afterthought

While finalising the script, already answering some questions after having sub-mitted a first version, and thus with some time having passed since first taking up the work, it becomes clear to me that than pandemics helped to highlight part of the polity-virus but even without such an extreme and extremely manifest threat the Precarity of Society as System Crisis is sadly obvious.

Sure, Corona is still occasionally issued as threat, new variants striking—but by and large the pandemics are not a topic on the political agenda anymore. This does not mean that the socio-economic consequences are solved. Going together with other major economic crises and hazards small shops are under severe pressure; social provisions and services—be it health care, child care, education and also the capacities of municipal administrations—are overburdened and even standard obligatory acts are hugely delayed, offices closed for the public, allowing staff to catch up with the growing piles of files; the housing situation a matter of serious concern—and the government trying to cushion the problems by occasional grants to relieve the burden on certain groups.

The hopes for a fundamental change, however, burst like soap bubbles: While climate activists are blocking roads and motor highways, highlighting the dangers of global warming, asking for roundtables and negotiations, they are in many cases criminalised and/or met by aggressive measures. At the same time, pri-vate transport is fostered, now focusing on electromobility while negotiating the reform of public transport and the relevant pricing systems are suffering from the same weakness as they had been shown above in relation to Covid 19. In Berlin, after a successful referendum I support of the socialisation of the property of large housing corporations according article 15 Basic Law, there are again and

P. Herrmann, *Pandemics as Matter of a System Crisis,* Prekarisierung und soziale Entkopplung – transdisziplinäre Studien, https://doi.org/10.1007/978-3-658-43450-2_12

again new hurdles erected: socialisation cannot become real, if it goes beyond ruinous payment of selective relief funds ...

The emperor's new dress showing that the ruler is still trapped in the structures of the small princedoms. He only reacts with fear, but without strategy, to the fact that the people have turned their backs on him. In the 'positive' case, it is addicted to individualism and withdraws more or less depressively into itself or the family as own little princedom; in the negative case, it follows the populist pied pipers (although such an allusion to the fairy tale of the *Pied Piper of Hamlin* needs some qualification).—Still, a certain loyalty to the system is, of course, still maintained by the fact that the powers—be it in business, government and the mass media—still succeed in building up an external enemy. If, though, today's challenges are global, not knowing any borders, it would be wiser to focus on real cooperation.

The True Virus Hiding Behind Covid19—an Adjunct Essay

13

This section had been elaborated in the early months of the pandemic, presenting very much a personal review of 'living in two worlds'. By and large the text is unchanged, apart from some minor alterations, primarily a matter of language (spelling, grammar …). It is more impressionistic, though important as contribution to the discussion of human rights and precarity, offering the possibility of contextualisation. This—and the need for contextualisation—is not least an argument against (a) formal assessments and (b) a view that is—primarily or even solely—geared towards the situation of individuals. Importantly, talking about Human Rights, means to talk structurally about social rights insofar humans are social beings. Obviously, social is here not limited to the understanding of communication, solidarity and/or mutual support. Instead, we are dealing with a complex concept, referring to the social as 'outcome of the interaction between people (constituted as actors) and their constructed and natural environment. Its subject matter refers to people's interrelated productive and reproductive relationships. In other words, the constitutive interdependency between processes of self-realisation and processes governing the formation of collective identities is a condition for the social and its progress or decline.' (van der Maesen/Walker 2012: 260) This means as well that precarity can only be understood as a structural change concerning the entire socio-economic setting—the living and working conditions of individuals and/or the emergence of a precariat. Instead, we are concerned with the possible (re-)structuration of society, a matter that must be seen as state of an existing system reaching its limits, though the alternative not yet being visible.

P. Herrmann, *Pandemics as Matter of a System Crisis,* Prekarisierung und soziale Entkopplung – transdisziplinäre Studien, https://doi.org/10.1007/978-3-658-43450-2_13

13.1   Introduction

Just to be clear from the outset: thinking biology, medicine and the like are as exact science impeccable, without errs, is hugely contestable. But this is not the topic—it only deserves mention as some definitely competent people stated that without downplaying the dangers, they should not be exaggerated and, for Corona there is surely something to be said about the virus being very much 'holder of its own passports'.

13.2   My Life With the Corona Virus—The Early Days

Short time before the Spring-Festival-holidays 2020, I faced some difficulty at the checkout of a supermarket—Biyu, another customer helped me …, thorough knowledge of language definitely helps. Then, bidding farewell, she said: I am so sorry that you experience the country now, the virus doesn't allow real Spring Festival Mood. Strangely enough it seemed that she worried more about me missing out, than her own 'loss'. Every little makes a difference—I remember one Christmas day, when I lived in Ireland, a nearly county-wide power cut making it impossible to 'live Christmas with the traditional turkey'—more worrying than anything else. This is not to say that the Irish aren't hospitable or less hospitable than Chinese people. But it still may point on a rather meaningful difference between East and West (this as any other categorisation must be taken with care !!): There is generally a more pragmatic orientation to be found in China— call it resignation, subordination or you also may call it freedom, of which one definition says that it is the 'insight into necessity'.

13.3   Visiting Europe Again

I had to go to Europe for a conference—it had been end of February 2020. Arriving at the airport in Munich—the flight had been hugely delayed—I had been asked by the officer at the border control how things had been. I mentioned heavy storms, reason for the delay of about one day, not really thinking about the virus as everything in China had been smoothly organised along the said line: insight into necessity. After a notion of puzzlement, the officer brought me back into the wider weird reality, talking about the lack of awareness, the non-existence of caution: 'We just have gloves for protection—actually we have them permanently, if there is a virus or not.' At this stage I had been myself not thinking seriously about the extent of the threat: after a few days in Munich, I went to the conference in Russia, moving from there to a meeting held by the European Academy of Science and Arts in Austria.[1] The plan had been to return from there to China, where in actual fact I have had already for the next day a connecting flight, bringing me to another conference. More or less last minute I received the info that all flights had been cancelled and there would not be any way to return in the foreseeable future.

At least I had been lucky, being able to accommodate myself in Berlin …. What I saw those days had been just the opposite of freedom, understood as insight into necessity: first, complete ignorance, of course suggesting that there is a problem in China, but still laughing at me, who had been at this stage one of the very few people, wearing a protective mask. This changed soon, reactions being increasingly protective—here protective is just another word for hostile; the reaction had been reminding of stepping hastily into a chicken barn, exaggerating reactions instead of a calm, systematic approach.

Some examples, impressions. And as valuable—and a bit entertaining—as they are, a systematic analysis, perhaps under the title of *The Virologist's Socio-Political Compass,* would be valuable for developing global responsibility and rights-based approaches as crisis management.

13.4   Oh Folks, Remain Realist …

Definitely, it is for us in China a kind of nightmare-situation: the threat, the insecurity, the psychological strain and also simply the inconvenience and thus physical strain: shops being closed, villagers deciding quarantine-ing themselves and people just accepting, staying calm and cooperating. And then ….—the German news magazine DER SPIEGEL (6/1.2.2020) coming up with a title-page showing a man in a kind of war-gear, even with a typical gas mask, stating: 'Corona Virus MADE IN CHINA. When globalisation becomes a deadly threat.'

Sorry, for me it is not only sending a wrong message, but it is also simply tasteless … 'when globalisation is becoming a deadly danger', with the implicit accusation that China is in an offensive mood …, I suppose globalisation as

---

[1] By the way, a rather intimidating event, marked by unbelievable ignorance of basic democratic principles: the then president showing himself as example par excellence for the old white men: ignorance paired with stubbornness, senility, careerism, overstretched self-esteem, pretending to stand above any god [from my point of view, not believing in the existence of any God, he has to be classified, following the terms of logic, as negative existence.

deadly threat should be said when it comes to Rana Plaza in Bangladesh, though mind: again not produced there, in India ...; and so many other similar incidents could be added...

Indeed, there is something else made in China—the other day I received a message from a former student of mine—from the time when I had been teaching economics. We are still in touch, and I sent him a message, just the hello and how are you and take care—here is part of the answer I received in return:

Not only protecting myself, also protecting people around me. Ordered nearly 1800 face masks from Japan last week and looking forward to receive them. Going to sell them at original price with a limit number per person and donate revenue from selling them. Purchased 2 kg of 'hand desinfektionsgel' from Germany for my parents.

Now, I would not even be surprised if *les boches* claim that this is 'German benevolence'...............

'Hello, I thank you for this letter and the assurance of solidarity from the German side.' While searching for this mail-address of the BS, I also see the reference to the naturally welcome wish for respectful cooperation. Germany and the AA (foreign ministry) cannot be everywhere and control everything. But I must confess that such a tasteless cover picture, like the one of the Spiegel, simply shakes me. The experience that I make, living in China, lets me see with my German passport such an insult with shame and anger.

Der Spiegel is not the German press, and I can only hope that this is the exception to the rule of reporting. Looking at this 'naughtiness' of the seal with criticism and rejection, a rebuke from the AA would certainly be compatible with the freedom of the press, because this is equally a matter of responsibility in reporting.

With kind regards

Peter Herrmann

13.5   Every Little Counts—The Common Good

Finally, with 14 h delay, I left the Empire of the Middle on the 9th of February—I use this old-fashioned reference to mark the ongoing mystification of China, but also other Asian countries: in the West there is often a strange way of ..., well, call it respect for the unknown, the exotic. And as exotic as anything unknown is, a new version of 'the magic' appeared to me, walking from the shuttle train to the final passport control: the 'magic' of a futurist scenario:

Please, walk slowly—temperature measurement in progress
Compliance again, very likely everybody saying I do not want to be infected and I do not want to infect anybody else—sure this measurement is not the proper medical one in the strict sense …, but *every little helps.* Big Brother as good friend—let's take it pragmatically. And of course, every control has different sides. This is what I mentioned earlier, completing a questionnaire from the airport security, amongst others containing the questions:

1) Have you ever have had temperature?
2) Did you feel exhausted recently?

I guess even every toddler did have temperature and then: in connection with the delay of the flight I had been chased across the airport for a couple of times—consider that I'm not trained olympionique, consider as well that I'm not the youngest anymore, it seems quite natural that I had been exhausted. *Every little helps …*, and *every little needs attention,* even the smallest thing, including precise wording of questions. All this shows that there is always the 'human factor', leaving us with some errors of a special nature: Formal approaches are applied, assumptions are made and the best and probably the only thing we can do is moving on, accepting the four fundamental notions:

1. Common sense is—not always, but often—a sound guide for our action and activities and behaviour
2. Though we may often feel alone—seemingly a characteristic of modern societies—we are never alone; thus, any kind of complex situation and process needs to be explored from different sides, not only considering what is self-evident for ourselves (think about it: you see something that is 'yellow'; your friend sees the same thing but does not see it as yellow but as 'in a very bright colour'—you may easily end up in some misunderstanding).
3. Not least: communication is decisive—society had been characterised by various terms: society as theatre, as leisure society, court society, welfare society, and of course as industrial society, service society, class society, middle class society. It is Niklas Luhmann's merit to have introduced the term communication society, however, he understood communication in such a way that …, ehem, there had not been any people left: communication in his understanding had been a process without subjects (there is nothing wrong if you do not understand this 'autopoietic process'—it cannot be understood; it has a bit of swimming in a lake without getting wet). I propose another hyphen-society may be a *court-room society,* the

latter understood as place where justice is negotiated by applying a specific language, one that is necessarily both, precise and disputatious, neutral and strictly goal-oriented.

4. This way the *every little helps,* combined with the *every little needs attention* is joined by a third pillar, namely *everybody has an important role to play.*

Thus, the Kantian categorical imperative –

A. Act only according to that maxim whereby you can, at the same time, will that it should become a universal law (this is the wording from Kant's *Grounding for the Metaphysics of Morals* from 1785 (Kant, 1785), later he used slightly different formulations)

applies, but needs to be enhanced:

B. Act only according to that maxim whereby you can, at the same time, will that your action and activity is well interwoven and coordinated with the action and activities of others

and

C. Act only according to that maxim whereby you can, at the same time, will that the result is one that can prove validity in the future.

And the expert may justifiably feel tempted to see some Rawlsian *veil of ignorance* at play (see Rawls 2001).

Leaving the funny (not to say ridiculous) aspects of obviously (and also seemingly) unreasoned questions aside, there is another, serious issue, not least in perspective of rights to be raised: we are always caught between highly standardised means, possibly applied in a mechanical way and the need for what had been frequently called the *struggle for law,* that is the dispute and human empathy to elaborate a solution that is just, meaning that is appropriate to the situation. In more common terms we are looking at the tension between legality and justice (and those who studied law will of course remember the seminars on the different takes on 'ought' and 'is').

This section may be concluded by the most crucial point, arising from what had been said so far: at the very core we are dealing with the common good, and importantly this stands at the beginning—as such it is one of the interpretations of Marxist thinking, expressed in two frequently quoted sentences:

'Men make their own history, but they do not make it as they please; they do not make it under self-selected circumstances, but under circumstances existing already, given and transmitted from the past', standing at the beginning of *The Eighteenth Brumaire* (Marx 1852: 103).

And in the *Introduction to the Outline of the Critique of the Political Economy*

'The human being is in the most literal sense a ζῷον πολιτιχόν [political animal], not merely a gregarious animal, but an animal which can individuate itself only in the midst of society'.

It would be problematic to see this as superiority of the social—such interpretation presupposes the social as 'reification of its own', arising from nowhere—like a *deus ex machina*. However, this common good is nevertheless of special—quasi-superior—character, as it is source and objective of acting individuals; take (a) simple issues as language (needed to speak with somebody else, something that is shared), (b) more complex issues as common sense and morals (yes, something you share) or (c) highly elaborated systems as the regulative body (or call it civil code and related legislation) of a country or the trans- and international system—and remember: crossing the street, buying a tiny commodity or making a present ....

all these are, despite and with their purely moral, human, humane and emotional dimension, *legal acts*. Highlighting the crucial meaning of the social—for instance in form of the common good—gains at present some special relevance as in the context of COVID19, one of the leading online gazettes on EU-affairs laments in its BRIEF *(Stam, without date)* that '[t]he swiftly-spreading coronavirus forces all of us to take a reality-check and face the ugly truth. It also forces us to adapt and change our behaviour for the common good. Because this is what it is all about. This is what is at stake.' This statement—and the then following reference to 'disruption' caused by the virus, is remarkable, showing the Western (under)valuation of the public good: peripheral, related to emergencies, the last resort. With some good will, one can see it as slip—an argument of bad taste brought forward by one of the many unsettled journalists. However, for me, looking at EU policies over the years, in particular the debate of services of general interest, there cannot any doubt that there is little appreciation of the common good as general standard: everything is geared to individuals, looking for their own, personal benefit.

Doesn't this connect nicely with the argument I brought forward, when addressing the international Human Rights Conference in Changsha in December2019 (Herrmann, December 2019), an argument that is widely discussed, often as matter of a fourth generation of human rights—here I would put it under the heading of human rights (also) as right of humanity, not (only) of individuals.

A brief link may be established: while the issue is here discussed on the meta-level of human rights, it equally boils down to various concrete issues, not least the increasing precarity of Western societies and the working and employment situation emerging under the pressure of the developed capitalist system, which Branko Milanovic sees as *'Capitalism alone' (Milanovic 2019)*. Also in respect of (living and) working conditions, including the design of employment contracts, we are confronted with the need to deal with the question 'how do the working and employment conditions' shape society, what are the costs and benefits of any regulation for society (obviously, of course, the cost of ill-health in case of insufficient security, monetary cost also for public health systems but also as cost of social quality.

13.6   Freedom and the Control of the Individual that Lacks Insight Into Necessities

Of course, mentioning 'common goods' remains abstract, as long as we do not connect it to concrete forms of social and societal processes. The same is true, if we look at anthropological patterns, usually claiming to be constant, characterising human behaviour independent of socio-historical formations. Remaining on this general level, it is probably fair to say that two tensions guide human beings in their behaviour and acting: The one is the tension between the *Ought-To-Be* and the _Is;_ the other is the tension between the *individual will* and *societal dynamics*. However, making any anthropological reference must acknowledge that it is always about an anthropology that is specifically shaped by the concrete formation that serves as 'frame' and 'network of rails' *(see Herbert Marcuse 1966)*.

Taking this as point of departure, we can see that another issue is about security and problem management—understood as individual and as well as a collective issue. However, such general statement needs to be clarified by establishing a concrete understanding of the different points in question. These are in particular the understanding of *security,* the definition of the **collectivity**, and the understanding of *responsibility*. Against this background the following will highlight some sets of norms and behaviour, allowing a tentative classification [the following may be a justifiable simplification when it comes to different ways in which the crisis is encountered and managed]—in some respect we can see this as reflection of different understandings of the common good.

- *La Vita e Bella* – even if circumstances changed to the worst. Central is the notion *Nessun Problema* – no problem. First, any expectation that comes along as a restriction is refuted, then fearfully accepted but only on a superficial level. The pattern is actually well-known from intercultural studies with—amongst others—the following traits:
  - proxemics *(relevant is what is close to me,* not what is at distance)
  - denial—why should I worry …, it is not me, it is not here (like the child, for whom the parent seemingly does not exist anymore as soon as he/she is around the corner)
  - chronemics *(time as 'wild ocean', things overlapping and everything has to be dealt with the second it occurs* instead of seeing time as chronologically occurring processuality, like the linen hung up to dry, one after the other …)—which translates into dealing with things as they occur, without any strategic consideration, as in the case of the virus: its coming had been foreseeable but remained ignored until it actually showed up for some time
  - kinesics (most part of communication is non-verbal, its interpretation very much depending on tacit knowledge, *a pattern that is emphasised, using strong gestures and an expressive body language, appearing to the outsider as eccentric*/something that is not explicitly 'used', the person him/herself by and large not being aware of it, reserved, hiding behind a mask of neutrality).

How does it translate into the way the Corona-crisis is encountered? Taking from some recent communication with my former fellow-citizens (I lived a couple of years in Rome, the city that claims to host the Holy Grail of western culture): initially, seeing some shops closed, panic showed in eyes and words, feeling like being innocently imprisoned: not being allowed to visit the coffee bar (for 'us Italians' only a matter of minutes, but as essential as the boring blue suit, standard dressing for the standard Italian gentlemen), not being able to meet neighbours and friends for a chat and making up rumours … .—all under the veil of innocence, as Catholicism, the quasi-state-religion, is about exactly this: escapism as escape into the here and now, as a friend says: people are having more time for family, to look after themselves … and they are singing from the balconies and rooftops.—All this sounds nice …, until we are getting aware of some bitter facts: the health services are collapsing under unbearable pressure, mismanagement and the lack of an early coordination of intervention.

Pestalozzi pointedly saw the reality behind the search for real solution, speaking of the

„Auslöschen der bürgerlichen Tugend durch den Trug einer wahrheitsleeren Sittlichkeit und ihr Verscharren des Rechts in die Mistgrube der Gnade für das zu erklären, was es wirklich ist.'—'*Extinguishing civic virtue through the deception of an empty morality, and declaring its burial of law in the dung-pit of grace for what it really is.'* (Pestalozzi)

Being a country that depends economically to a large extent on tourism, it is—at first glance—of course the best to deny as long as possible. And sadly—though not limited to this country—the strategy followed the principle 'it had not been me': looking for the origin in order to think about preventive measures is of course appropriate; however, to point with the finger on 'the bad boys' (it is suggested that the virus arrived from France and Germany, saying that both countries did not take any security measures) is another thing. In a nutshell, it is what Francesco, a friend, said many years ago, when I criticised the result of the elections. His reply: *'Certo, Berlusconi è una vergogna. Ma in realtà nessuno si preoccupa di quelo che fa il governo centrale. Noi italiani facciamo quello che ci piace fare. [Sure, Berlusconi is a disgrace. But actually nobody bothers what the central government does. We Italians do what we like to do.]'* – And indeed, both are common: the romantic scene of people standing on rooftops or balconies; singing like Luciano Pavarotti, acting like Totò or Sophia Loren…, and feeling like Romeo and Juliette; the common joy—or should I say: the joy of common action—also now and also as expression of solidarity as for instance the virtual choir that is dedicated to the medical workers (https://youtu.be/VubAWDQ3gco); and on the other hand the extremely poor, neglected and self-neglecting—the ugly, not even waiting for the beast, knowing that it will be at most the helpless helper, more likely the police or the fellow citizen who denies their right to be fellow citizen. It may be taken as recurrence of those medieval times: ten young people enjoying themselves in a retreat, mutually entertaining by their narrations, while the ordinary people had been victims of the black death. Boccaccio's well-known *Il Decamerone* (古腾堡计划中收录的), the well-known outcome, enjoyed by many even today; aiming on forgetting the suffering of the many, wiping it away—today as in those days.

- *Alles im Griff* – all well controlled and ordered, also a matter of individual freedom—but European freedom has different faces, the German version is about well-ordered life. The country is for good reason known for law and order—the country of poets and thinkers *(in German: Dichter und Denker)* being at the very same time the country of judges and hangman *(in German: Richter und Henker)*. There are definitely huge advantages of federalism, in principle realising by and large the catholic notion of subsidiarity, suggesting that decisions should be taken as near as possible to the people who are concerned—and actually they should be taken by the people. But we find also the re-interpretation of this principle in the light of the protestant work ethics as presented by Max Weber: work hard for your own benefit, which will be rewarded in the after-life—or as the saying goes *'every man for himself, and God for us all'* (admittedly a slightly obscured presentation of a relatively complex ideology). All this sounds reasonable and attractive, doesn't it? However, there is definitely a miscalculation when it comes to Corona:

While seemingly something that occurs in multitude, there is only ONE virus: instead of looking for ONE answer, in Germany every Land ('county') is looking for its own answer: in some there is more or less business as usual, only large public events are not taking place, in others the County-Government announced the state of emergency, some issues are up to the decision by the municipalities ...—and in any case, the state of fear is a reaction of the virus and the lack of political and administrative security. Taking up the patterns presented above for Italy, it looks somewhat different for a country like Germany:

- proxemics *(relevant is as well what is close to me,* not what is at distance
- denial—why should I worry ..., it is not me, and it is not here (but not like the child, for whom the parent seemingly does not exist as soon as he/she is around the corner; instead, *it is about the illusion of protestant work ethics: being industrious, not chasing up for the joyful life but being convinced of 'standing above evil')*
- chronemics (time as 'wild ocean', things overlapping and everything must be dealt with the second it occurs—here this wild ocean *is chronologically ordered, like the linen hung up to dry, one after the other ...* – this translates into dealing with things not as they occur, but in a strategic way, ...— elaborating a plan, consolidating the plan, coordinating it with the different countries, coming to the conclusion that such coordination is not possible, revisiting the plan on the regional level ... this sounds more than ridiculous; and while the advantages of federalism are not completely denied, it is suggested that it is not a pattern that can claim general validity (the reform of the German language *[Dittrich, 2016]* at the end of the last century showed indeed such a pattern of taking decisions, recalling them again to take them again in one of the Laender, but not the other etc,.—meaning also a huge material loss. Huge losses are currently also accepted by orienting along the lines of herd immunisation, without any further backing—it is a Darwinist mechanism, following the principle of the survival of the fittest.

The presumption is that it is necessary that approximately 60 to 70% of the population needs to be infected so that one can speak of immunity being reached—allowing this means to allow at the very same time a high mortality rate: especially older people, young children, people living under unhealthy conditions (substandard accommodation, homeless people …) these are most vulnerable groups, most likely victims paying with their lives.

- kinesics (most part of communication is non-verbal, its interpretation very much depending on tacit knowledge, a pattern that is emphasised, using strong gestures and an expressive body language, appearing to the outsider as eccentric – *here this is not explicitly 'used', the person him/herself is by and large not aware of it, reserved, hiding behind a mask of neutrality*).

At some stage then, this neutrality and remaining individual freedom turns into its opposite: the fear if one behaves correctly, if the relevant government (though one may not know which one is relevant in the case in question) made an announcement of which one is not aware, the fear also of the other: isn't everybody potential host of the virus: the other and oneself? It is not the *bellum omnium contra omnes* (war of all against all), Thomas Hobbes was talking about—or perhaps it is: at least the very moment one stands in front of the empty shelves, the milk being sold out, the moment juicy lemons are sold out and one has to buy the more expensive ones, not really suitable for freshly pressed juice …, facing the empty shelves, one has the idea that there could be another virus at play, the virus of fear, which is itself a hiding place, the real name being the 'left-alone-you-must-fight-for-yourself-virus'. Feudalism, in its absolutist version, had been about the king, announcing *'l'état c'est moi'*. The anti-feudal revolution, at least part of it, resulted in making—at least seemingly—everybody king, everybody defining him/herself as owner of the common good, boldly claiming as individual what actually belongs to the community—and one may feel alone, though standing in the middle of countless others.

Now, the latter has to be qualified as many are staying at home—being told to do so or escaping into the apparent security of 'the home being a castle'; all this may well be about the revival of the family, mutual support and public responsibility: on the latter, after years of seriously deconstructing the public health system, the UK plans investment in the health sector; the head of the *Deutsche Städte- und Gemeindebund (German Federation of Cities and Communities)* stating *'We are currently becoming a little more considered about whether it is really economic efficiency that is so decisive, whether it is not necessary to say: We are going to maintain certain hospitals, even in the wider terrain.' (Landsberg,*

March 11ᵗʰ, 2020; translation P.H.). And the family? According to some sources the lack of structuration of the day, living together on limited space, not being used to lively children and the like can often cause domestic violence *(domestic violence*—https://www.msn.com... *).*

- EUropean unity—how should it work if unity does not work on the national level and between the member states. In actual fact, lack of coordination and cooperation is in several instances the better option—better at least than competition, hostility and envy. However, the latter is by far not uncommon. Even in those circles, we call commonly enlightened and aware about responsibility, we find critique that may well be founded, appears as hostile afront, brought forward emotionally instead of searching for common solutions in solidarity. Of course, this is in some way understandable; however, it is surely not helpful. Just a few examples may show what is meant:
  - The Italian South Tyrolian tourist industry, severely hit by the corona-bust, complains that in the German North Rhine Westphalia more cases can be counted—many other cases of shaming and blaming could be listed. The mentioned case is, however, especially meaningful as it is about reviving patterns of nationalism that reach far back. Isn't this a clear sign, showing that the discussion is not about human lives but about political interests of nationalism and protectionism?
  - Referring to Italy another time is just a matter of 'bing-MSN-random news'—the browser setting of the computer, unchanged after purchase. Having a look at one of the headlines ...—well, a matter of taste and I would personally say the presentation of the more or less complete lockdown by the Prime Minister shows a pathos that is close to crudity.
  - Primarily an issue between the United States of America and China, we find also the European Union playing a role in the trade war: mainly the rise of China is seen as threat, although one should be more precise and speak of geopolitics and a global trade war: the People's Republic of China is indeed the most successful of a group of countries that is increasingly a threat to the so-called developed world. Sure, a manifold of issues is at stake: the so-called Boomerang-effect, the questionable Rostowian model, the debate concerning the explanatory reach of quantitative approaches (in particular the questioning of GDP) towards measuring progress are just a few. Leaving all this aside, it is of interest that the hegemonic position of 'the West'—the USA, the EU and the EU-USA—is questioned. While China is one of the main 'push points', countries as Brazil and not least international cooperative efforts as BRICS and 'the Belt' must also be seen

as perceived threat. In this light, Covid19 is a welcome opportunity to argue against China, and to propose even 'China virus' as name—we see only slowly the awareness that cause and dealing with epidemics and mass diseases is something that needs to be approached globally *(an interesting course from Yale-university can be found here: HIST 234 ....—though already from Spring 2010, it did not lose anything of its meaning).* – It is surely a bit trite, but there is some truth in what supposedly Blaise Pascale, theologian, physicist, mathematician, physicist, and inventor, living in the seventeenth century, said: 'All men's miseries derive from not being able to sit in a quiet room alone.' Shall we take it as variation of the insight that man is a social being?—Summarising and in short: not competition and blame, but cooperation and understanding should be at stake.

– Sure, there is more to it, but can we expect citizens behaving rational and considerate, if their political leaders aren't? At stake is, indeed, the long-term hegemonic notion that characterises 'Western Modernity'. There is, of course, the danger of throwing the baby out with the bathing water, denying the progressive side of the development. However, experiencing the negative side in such a concentrated form as I do now, makes me probably feeling for the first time deeply what this Europeaness is about: I am not talking about the short-term issue, namely the reaction to the pandemic and its management. It is a mindset that shapes history in the longue durée, the temps des événements and as well the time spanning between these poles *(see Braudel 1987: 30).* It is a common and firm floor, providing sufficient ground for erecting differently featured superstructures. In the present context superstructure is not understood in the traditional Marxist sense; instead, reference is made to the theory of regulation, here put forward in an extended and elaborated form. The core consists of the accumulation regime, the life regime, the mode of regulation and finally the mode of living. In a nutshell and in a more or less casual formulation they can be defined as follows:

the accumulation regime is the way in which we make money and spend it for (re-)production

the life regime presents the fundamental pattern of production and consumption in the perspective of classes and social groups

the mode of regulation can be understood as the framework and the rail system, supporting and limiting the processes of accumulation

finally we arrive at the way in which individuals translate the general opportunities and restrictions into their real life on a daily basis.

Taking this as framework, we find individualism, short-termism and localism being centre-staged by systems and individuals alike. This is in the European and more general western debate today frequently reflected as part and parcel of neoliberalism. While it is in some respect a valid reference, it is easily forgotten that neoliberalism itself is a complex and differentiated system. One important aspect can be seen in the fact that we find on the national level and equally in the European Union patterns of centre-periphery-relationships, as they had been analysed and elaborated by Immanuel Wallerstein. It is this constellation where we find mutual dependencies, that make an escape nearly impossible. Individual behaviour can hardly be changed due to system requirements; change of the system is equally impossible due to the endurance of individual behaviour. Equally, there is the blockage between the accumulation regime and the life regime on the one hand and the mode of regulation and the mode of living on the other hand. The complexity is furthered by the tension between the two different regimes and between the two modes (*En passant,* underestimating this complexity and its political-economic grounding is the problem with—in tendency—subjectivist approaches, that focus on a supposed imperial mode of life without reflecting on the complexity of transponders, responders and transponders— an approach that is brought forward by Ulrich Brand and Markus Wissen and their conceptualisation of the imperial mode of living).

One further point remains to be mentioned: all these examples are not least a matter of a certain arrogance of the Western countries towards Asia and in particular towards China. This is about the underlying assumption of the 'advanced countries' being advanced in their cultural development, their ability to avoid catastrophes like this and to deal with them in the supposedly unlikely case of their occurrence. Although very critical about the politics in China, Verena Kreilinger and Christian Zeller state:

> *Many of them also assumed that our rich countries, with their excellent technical infrastructure, would be able to cope with such a challenge. Some of them still do, which is similar to the behaviour of the so-called 'climate deniers'. This reflects a complete failure to recognise the dynamics of the spread of the virus, the limited capacity of our health infrastructure and the economic and social consequences of this crisis.*

(Kreilinger/Zeller, 21.3.2020; Translation P.H.)

At least since the middle of March 2020 we find some European awareness; this is, however, not a matter of coordination. Instead, it is about the development of a common understanding of the supposed need defined by the European accumulation regime. Verena Kreilinger and Christian Zeller again, suggest:

In this article we highlight the serious failures of European governments and the EU in particular. Deliberate decisions, misjudgements and omissions led to Europe becoming the epicentre of the corona pandemic. Governments and the EU are not able to take the measures necessary for the health and well-being of the population. They cannot do so because they are subject to the primacy of capital accumulation and competitiveness. Instead of making the necessary cuts in all sectors of the economy that are not necessary for social care, they prefer to let an unspecified number of people die.

(Ibid.)

As said, it is not just the reaction on the pandemic. Indeed, it is perhaps the first time that I really feel Europeanness—a mindset that shapes history in the longue durée showing its exclusivity clearer than usually: exclusive also meaning exclusion.

Earlier it had been already said that this is founded in and leads to individualism, translating into egoism and egocentrism, presentism as orientation on short term periods, localism in terms of 'reachable space' and finally exclusionism as matter of externalisation. It seems to be fair to see the focus of the entire—Western? Modern?—mindset oriented on the supposed compatibility of defining the common goods by individuals, resulting also in a strange utilitarian understanding of one's own life.

Tinder, one of the so-called social networks is an example par excellence— what *Uber* and *Didier* are for 'ride-sharing', is tinder for partner- ..... -search: 'use & enjoy & drop', just as you like ... - ops, just as I like. The critique here is not based on any puritan attitude; it is not questioning changing sexual partners. At stake is ..., well, even this terminology of things 'being at stake': we are permanently creating ourselves not as personalities but as stakes, 'items on a scale' *(see also Herrmann, December 2018);* and paradoxically, we always feel or pretend to feel that we are serving and performing—somebody or something, thus justifying the claim to have some time, space for oneself, allowing some kind of retreat.

Most obviously the incongruence—between and within the nation states— results in different national, regional social 'performances', different with specific emphasis, related to religious festivities, specific national or regional experiences etc., though (nearly) never reaching a real collective identity, something for which we even lack a clear term. And what is togetherness as matter of the EU-member states? On the 26th of March, the EU-summit proves its inability to act *'with one voice and in support of those who need it most' (see the European Council, 26th of March, 2020).* The decisive step had been postponed: a systematic support programme for the two European member states that are under the most severe pressure.—Having mentioned earlier the being and feeling 'really European', remembering the earlier involvement in these debates *(see Herrmann: Time ...)*, it shows another side of what it can mean that history is like a nightmare, determining our life: there seems to be no way out—and protest from within doesn't change anything; at most it ends in the inability to act.

Hannah Arendt proposed, that it is not cruelty that characterises tyranny but the destruction of the public political realm, the tyrant monopolises for himself (a claim based on supposed wisdom or craving for power), thus insisting that the citizen cares for the private realm, leaving it to him to look after the public realm *(paraphrased from Arendt 1958: 215)*. Of course, this is a wide and difficult field—organisations of the civil society are often referred to and equally often criticised as extension of the state and/or the ruling classes *(see already the critique by Robert Michels, concluding 1915 in his book on Political Parties, an iron law of large organisations: to be effective and influential they have to grow; but if they grow, they stagnate and bureaucratise—see Michels, 1915)*. If this is an iron law ...? In my PhD-thesis *(see Herrmann 1994)* I, argued against it ... but that is another topic. Here, coming back to Hannah Arendt, we know that latest since the 'Thatcher era' such sentence as hers would have to refer today to 'him/herself' and 'him/her'. And looking at the 'public', one issue comes especially these days to the fore, while they are often ignored and forgotten when the question of freedom is discussed: While it is at least at first glance easy to prove individual freedom or oppression, one random pick of a daily newspaper *(Neues Deutschland, March 13th, 2020)* should make us thinking: page 13 (reports from the Land Brandenburg) has an entire column, considering the difficulties of 'limiting public life' in the run of the corona crisis management, about half the page reports on violence of right/fascist forces, 1/3 reports on economic difficulties of public hospitals, not least due to recent cutbacks; half a column on new police equipment; page 14 then: a long article with photo (more than ½ page) on the difficulties to maintain child protection due to recent cutbacks; a short note on shortages to establish barrier-free access of public places; nearly one column on the need of emergency investment: public schools being in a disgraceful state; approximately a third of a page on a 'deal' between a small town and the successors of the last Hapsburg-emperor, promising the family a huge amount of money and a gain of reputation. And in the same line it should make us think that China and Cuba are now helping other countries, not least Italy—they are helping in a situation that is much worsened by previous cutbacks. A look at relevant data is alarming: According to World Bank, the development of the number of beds and the medical staff decreases, a clear indicator for the 'success' of neoliberal policies—a frightening development in the light of standards based on professional requirements.

Just so far—some impressions …—looking at expressions: I suppose it is fair to say that much of what we witness is the combination of at least four strands:

- The objective 'threat' given by the virus, and the lack of knowledge countering it;
- The 'national social character'
- The objective conditions, not least the material resources that determine the space of action
- The 'sensibility of governments', aiming on coherence of policy making and citizenry—we may speak of social (dis)harmony.

While this gives some approximation, the strict classification goes along the lines of containment, i.e. the intended limitation of the spread of the virus; mitigation, the 'flattening of the curve'; and finally herd immunisation, possibly to be translated into 'famishment of the virus' and it can also be translated into 'feed the virus until it is saturated and calms down'—of course, the weakest being especially sacrificed. Each strategy is, of course, based in a specific interest and while caution is needed (as it is with any synopsis), the following can be taken for a useful approximation (Tab. 13.1):

Well, it surely is for all of us a difficult situation; difficult to deal and cope with in different respect: the fear of some, the need to accept requirements that limit behaviour, the coping with physical distance which sometimes really comes across as social distance and of course for many the difficulties emerging from material cuts and/or bureaucratic requirements.

Still, there is perhaps a global trend—just a trend that is visible and that is presented here without any qualification, any valuation. 26th of March, I receive a mail, informing me of the death of Lucien Seve—a profound critical thinker, who passed away already on the 23rd. The first victim of the virus I personally know …. knew—and even if he had been already in the 90s …. The message to me has also a link to a French daily, the Huma. I open the page, follow also another link:

'Gérer les décès, les familles, je n'y suis pas préparée…' Le témoignage bouleversant d'Alice, infirmière en réanimation—'Managing deaths, families, I am not prepared for it …'—The overwhelming testimony of Alice, resuscitation nurse— an article reporting on the work of a 33-year old, but also on the hypocrisy of

Tab. 13.1 Strategies, Means and Goals - an International Comparison

Strategy	Measures	Main Goal	Examples
Containment	More or less strict control of movement; reducing economic activities on what is necessary	Human lives	China, South Korea
Mitigation	Control of movement, especially targeted ('vulnerable people') and reducing economic activities on necessities	Health care management	Several EU-member states
Herd immunisation	Limited control of movement, often based on appeals; reducing economic activities, while maintaining that 'we will use all means we can avail of to ensure that the ... economy will withstand this storm.' (v.d. Leyen, 12. März 2020)	'keep business going' + health care management + securing individual freedom	Germany

a political system that leaves workers and patients alone. A very personal statement, emotionally touching .... Later I am talking to a colleague from one of the universities in Berlin. He invites me to join one of the next days for a drink: the regular's table of the institute, I am affiliated with—he sends me later the details: a URL. I promise to join, it will be after a meeting with colleagues from China, Italy and South Africa, preparing an online conference for early April. Indeed, another world is already happening, a somewhat weird world of which we have to master the dangers, and develop the opportunities ...—together.

For us an old debate must be taken up, under changing conditions—and it is of interest again what we find in *Pashukanis' Selected Writings on Marxism and Law:*

'Comrade Stuchka, from our point of view, correctly identified the problem of law as a problem of a social relationship. But instead of beginning to search for the specific social objectivity of the relationship, he returned to the usual and formal definition—although a definition now influenced by class characteristics. In the general formula given by Stuchka, law figures not as a specific social relationship but, as with all relationships in general, as a system of relations which corresponds to the interests of the ruling class and which protects it with organized force. Accordingly, within these class boundaries, law as a relationship is indistinguishable from social relations in general, and Comrade Stuchka is therefore not in a position to answer Professor Reisner's venomous question:

how do social relationships become legal institutions, or how is law converted into itself?' (Pashukanisdfgh 1924: 61)

13.7   Grounding

Only time will show and possibly not even that: there are different sources claiming to be the first of the phrase: *I don't trust any statistics that I did not made up myself.* Statistics and supposed scientific analysis arrives at different results. Insulting since there are simple explanations—for instance there is a difference between figures for regions and entire countries; the figures may appear as huge difference in the overall result. As such, scientific results are used as means, guiding political decisions, working always as contest of different individual measures. Ed Snowden proposed already about 10 years ago an interesting framework, presented in a lecture series where he posed 10 questions. It may be worthwhile to reproduce them in full length here *(from* https://oyc.yale.edu/history/hist-234/lecture-12*):*

> ### 10 Questions on Diseases
> 'I have a sort of suggestion of maybe ten major questions that we ought to be thinking about with regard to diseases.
> The **first** major question, for any of the diseases we're talking about, was what's the total mortality and morbidity that's caused by the epidemic in question? The mortality, the total numbers of deaths. Morbidity, the total number of cases. That's an important factor that needs to be taken into account in assessing the impact of the epidemic. A **second** question has to do with a term we introduced long ago, a phrase, which was the case fatality rate. And a related question with that is, is there an effective therapy or means of prevention, or instead does a society experience the disease in feeling itself to be helpless, and physicians feeling the same?
> The case fatality rate is — we could call it the kill rate of a disease, the percentage of cases that terminate in death. And we know that, for example, in dealing with plague, one of the features of it — and Asiatic cholera as well — was a very high case fatality rate, of plague, fifty to eighty percent, cholera, something like fifty percent. At the other extreme, when we come to it, we'll see that influenza has a very high morbidity, but quite a low case fatality rate, and that's related, I think, to the impact

that that disease, influenza, has on society, which isn't associated with such terror as say plague or cholera. That's an important variable, the kill rate of the disease.

Another factor, a **third** question we need to ask, is what's the nature of the symptoms of the infectious disease in question? Are they particularly painful? Are they degrading, according to the norms of the time? And we've seen, for example, in dealing with plague and cholera that a major feature about them was that their symptoms were agonizing and dehumanizing. Clearly, as we turn to syphilis, its symptoms also were extremely important in the way that the disease was experienced. Tuberculosis, on the other hand — and we'll be looking at that — was seen, at the time, to make its sufferers more intelligent, more romantic, more beautiful in some sense, at least in the first half of the nineteenth century. So, that — what is the nature of the symptoms, is a crucially important question.

Another, **fourth** question, that I hope you'll bear in mind throughout the course, and in your review for the exercise this week, is the question, is this disease new, or is it familiar to the population? Familiar diseases tend not to be so terrifying. The population is also likely to have some degree of immunity to the disease, and the disease is likely, or may have, already mutated to become less deadly. Examples are the so-called diseases of childhood, like chickenpox, mumps and measles; normally relatively mild, but in populations to which they're newly introduced, they can be devastating.

A **fifth** question has to do with, what's the profile of the victims of the disease? Is this a disease that's an affliction of the young and the elderly; that is, experienced as a more normal course of a disease, in accord with society's expectations and past experience? Or does it instead strike down particularly those who are in the prime of life, thereby no longer seeming natural but as something extraordinary in the experience of the population? And it also means that the disease is likely to maximize its economic and financial impact, to be particularly destabilizing to a community. Cholera, in this regard, for example, was terrifying because of the way in which it seemed to afflict those who were the bulwarks of families and of communities.

A **sixth** question that's important: what's the class profile of the sufferers? What sorts of people in society are stricken with the affliction? Is this a disease of poverty, such as cholera is usually thought of? Or is it an affliction that strikes everyone, without particular reference to class or social and economic status, like influenza or syphilis, indeed?

A **seventh** important question is what is the mode of transmission of the disease? Is it transmitted person to person? Is it transmitted by contaminated food and water? Are vectors involved? Is it spread through the air by droplets? Is it spread by sexual contact? And clearly, I think we'll be arguing that the mode of transmission is really crucial, and in sexually transmitted diseases I think that that is fairly self-evident and a very important factor in the social impact of those diseases.

An **eighth** important question is whether the disease is fulminant in its course, or is it slow acting and a wasting disease? If we look, for example, at cholera, one of the features, and a striking one, is that it was one of the most fulminant of diseases. It would strike down a sufferer, and you could board a train and die before you reached your destination, as the disease ran its course that quickly through the human body. Or, on the other hand, is the disease one that takes years, perhaps even decades, to run its course? And an example of that, of course, would be tuberculosis or HIV-AIDS, in our own time.

A **ninth** important question we need always to bear in mind is how is the disease understood by the population that it's infecting? Is it seen as a punishment of God? Is it later on thought to be something that comes from the dangerous classes? Or later on, is it understood to be a microbial infection? And those ways in which the disease is understood have enormous impact on how the population reacts to the disease. A **tenth** variable is what's the duration of the epidemic? Influenza, for example, passes through a locality in a matter of weeks, normally. Cholera or plague tend to have epidemics that last for months. And tuberculosis, one might describe as an epidemic in slow motion that afflicts a community for a whole century or more.'

There is another dimension which I want to propose as eleventh question: it is about confronting people with the situation, the grounding that serves as foundation before deciding different measures and approaches to fight the spread of the virus. As subheading of this section 'Grounding' I propose 'what are we really talking about?' And I want to start by telling a little story—one that seems to be completely unconnected to the question of policies against the spreading of the virus and fighting a pandemic. Although not a fairy tale, it begins with *once upon a time.* So, once upon a time, after a workshop meeting in Brussels, I went with some colleagues to a pub. All three had been Swedish nationals, two of them native Swedes, one of them holding Swedish passport but having been raised in Macedonia. We have been talking about some business; the Swedish-Macedonian colleague had been all the time moving along with the rhythm of the music, that had been played in the background. After concluding an agreement on my future work for some time in Sweden, one of two Swedish Swedes, looking little bit sad, said:

> 'Look at her—she is relaxed, enjoying herself, expressing frankly her emotions. It's so different, compared with me: standing still like a rock, wearing a grey suit, a grey shirt and a grey tie and probably all this mirrored in a grey face. I simply cannot jump out of this.'

This story does not end with the phrase 'and they lived happily ever after'—although they were all very nice people. The different character was showing up in the following months while we worked together. The reason for telling the story is very simple: currently Sweden is occasionally celebrated for a very open and liberal approach when it comes to dealing with the virus. There seems to be no lockdown, businesses are continuing work as they did earlier, schools and kindergardens remained open …. And still, the spread of the virus, its victims, and the mystic number 'R' remained seemingly reasonably low. Such policies of containing the spread of the virus is then frequently compared with strict measures of containing people: at some stage, people in Ireland had not been allowed to go further than two km from their home; in Germany the situation had been one of 'loose lockdown', in the Mediterranean countries we find 'strict lockdowns' … - relevant are also differences in the speed of reaction: some countries more or less hesitant, waiting some time before they introduced even harsher measures … - now I could tell another story, reflecting a telephone call one of the last days, speaking to a Chinese friend who is still working in the UK but quit her job in order to return to China.

'There are many reasons …..'

Taking the many reasons together, thinking also of what I heard from other Chinese friends and colleagues the many reasons may be summarised by saying.

> 'you know, there's something about home …—there I do not feel lonely, I am well looked after and things are done when they need to be done.'

Sure, much of this is anecdotal, is based on statements of few individuals out of a population of nearly 1,425,528,764 Chinese people *(Population China—* https://www.worldometers.info ...*)* and as such should not be overestimated. Nevertheless, it may well be taken as reflection of the often highlighted 'we-society'—some forms of control, but performing two roles at the same time: limitation and protection, the *chaxugeju* providing a framework and security bed that defines the individual (comparable with the African ubuntu, i.e. the 'I am because we are'), so entirely different if compared with the west where the individual is not defined by relations but a self-contained entity, striving to be different from others, even unique and even independent from others. Still, in using such terms, we should never forget that the meaning may will be different to Western uses of the terms.

'Organizational principles are to a society what a grammar is to a language. The principles provide the structural framework for social action; they are intuitive and taken for granted; they are deeply embedded in people's worldviews, as well as in the society that people re-create every day.' (Hamilton /Zheng 1992: 19)

So, looking at societies, the relevant economies and legal systems, is always about understanding those parts that are known to everybody: the tacit knowledge, usually not appearing in the textbooks (as it seems to be of no relevance) and not talked about amongst those who live their life accordingly (as it is too obvious in its permanent presence).

It is about the Guanxi in China, the Christian bonds in Europe, the family ties ... - but this is exactly the point: while we find families everywhere, their meaning is completely different.

Coming back to politics of controlling the spread of the virus, one of the main issues of the debate is about containment policies. With a very broad brush, being aware of the danger of stereotyping (and re-producing stereotypes), the following can be said:

- Celebrating Sweden as example of a liberal answer to the pandemics is questionable as it starts from two premises that are standing against the common understanding of liberal: • it is (aside of being other things) a country that is highly bureaucratic, the country of men wearing grey suits, grey shirts and grey ties, not allowing themselves to express emotions—self-containment does not need external control; • it is a country that is highly advanced in respect of social provisions, modern working conditions including home-office and the like—so it is obviously not really a matter of finding new regulations for what is given already by existing regulations and tacit rules

- Supposedly Lenin once said that the Germans, storming a railway station during a revolution, would first buy a platform ticket: rule bound and in need of rules, like the Alsation, so often used as service dog by the German police .... And still, one of the rules, in very general terms, is a welfare system that is still 'advanced': elaborated, bureaucratic, altogether grounded in the idea of a unified system, expressed in the fact of having a somewhat all-encompassing, comprehensive social code, the 'book of social law' (Sozialgesetzbuch) [including unemployment insurance but excluding labour law]—comprehensive does not mean accessible for everybody although accessibility had been one of the reasons for the reform by which the different areas of relevant 'social legislation' had been brought together. Today we speak of one book of social law, which consists now of 12 volumes, and a further extension is planned for 2024. Rule-obedience is thus closely linked to an expertocratic system—including non-obedience where expert-reasoning is lacking.—This is surely one of the reasons behind the important role given to the Robert-Koch-Institute. Representative of the organisation that is specialised on virus research frequently say that they cannot decide—instead there are political decisions, whereas the RKI can only provide data on the basis of which political decisions are to be taken. Here, the problem is about finding a balance between the authoritarian (not least it means submissive) character and the enlightened 'liberal' bourgeois. As formulated on an earlier occasion in this series of reflections: the country of poets and thinkers *(in German: Dichter und Denker)* being at the very same time the country of judges and hangman *(in German: Richter und Henker)*.

> There is a side-line to this, where the two actually meet, creeping into daily life without being noticed: much of the poesy and thinking is a matter of appearance, not of essence—the market, with its essence of making profit, comes along and makes profit even of the emergency and health threat: mouth and nose masks, after they had been sold out, are back, now already as 'new normality': in fashionable designs they are available—the sellers asking for 'the little bit more', the little bit that individuals can afford for 'looking good', but society cannot afford to look after those in need (Fig. 13.1).

- *Non posso crederci - non siamo qui per divertirci, non siamo qui per il momento, per fare un respiro profondo per ammirare le bellezze e le ricchezze dell'antichità..., e noi stessi, la famiglia e bambini? Restrizioni ..... -* incredibile - I cannot believe it—aren't we here to enjoy ourselves, aren't we here for the moment, taking a deep breath to admire the beauties and wealth of

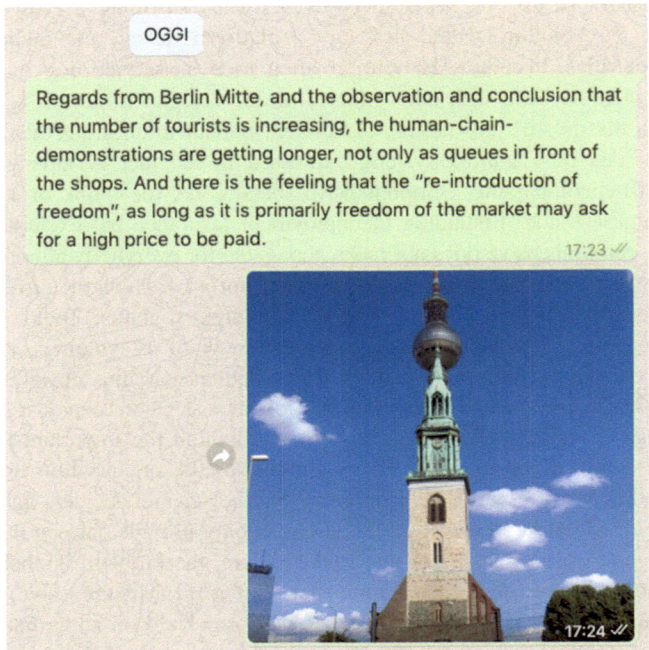

Fig. 13.1   Interests and Distribution of Power (own photo)

antiquity …, and ourselves, the family and children? Restrictions ….—unbelievable'—A torrent of words like this, and an emotionally based resistance, followed by cocooning, weirdly combined with an expressionist/exhibitionist and collectivist public performance of 'street balcony singing'. There is good reason behind extreme familiarism, regionalism, political extremism and short-termism characterising Italian politics—though 'electoral rule changes in the early 1990s turned Italy more towards majority governments' (Fig. 13.2)

- Prejudice? Maybe, though it may also be a reflection of the history of the United States of Northern America: a people that arrived there as a result of failing to claim their—mainly economic—freedom in their country of origin, welded together by religion, a commonly claimed right to occupy the country and expel the Indians and an extreme form of economic liberalism—the occupation of a vast area, the quasi tabula rasa in economic terms, where everything had to be started from the scratch and a kind of cultural new beginning (there

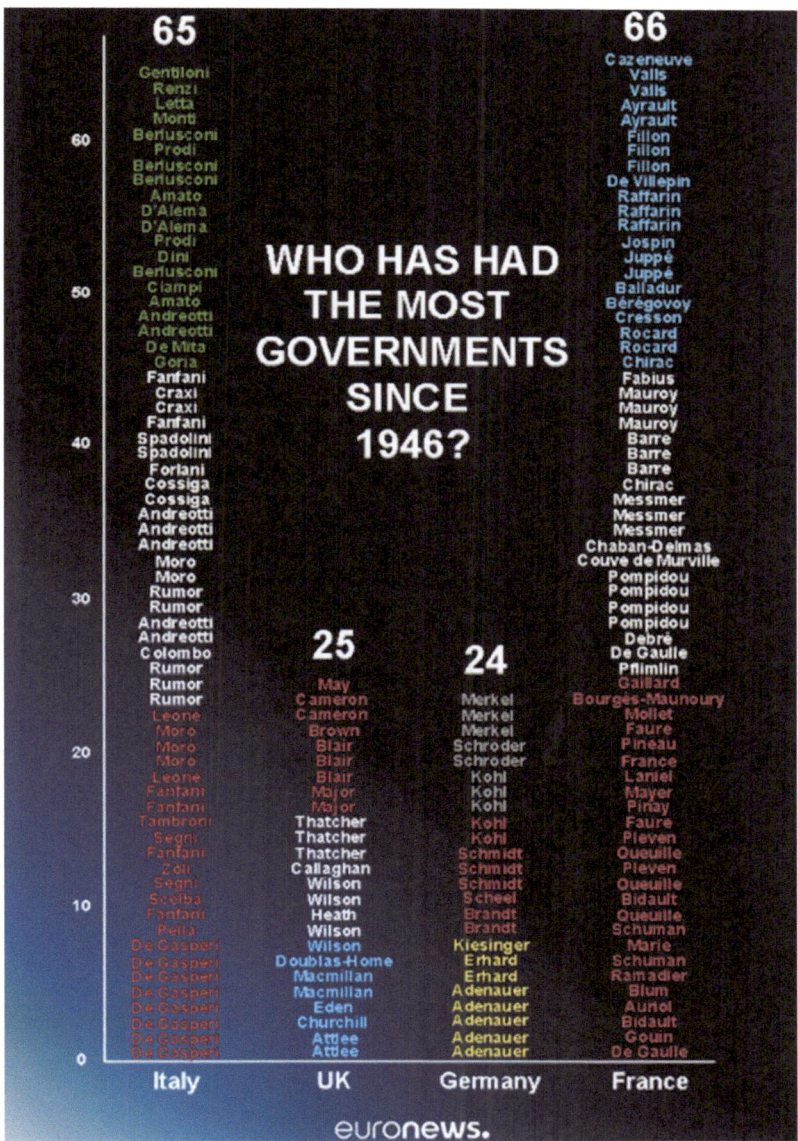

Fig. 13.2 Number of Changes of Governments in selected European Countries after 1949 *(Harris 2016)*

had not been anything they could build upon: in some way the own history had been rejected and the present culture of the Indians had been genocided),

(https://hemisphericinstitute.org/en/emisferica-14-1-expulsion/14-1-essays/the-border-s-crossed-us-too-the-intersections-of-native-american-and-immigrant-fights-for-justice-2.html#images-2; *05/07/2023*) (Fig. 13.3)

established the feeling of superiority, later elevated to a claim of world leadership, i.e. the role of a world gendarme.

What can a virus do to a people like this? How could God hurt a people that makes even a Muslim president a professing Christian? And yet: the flip side is that everyone must be seen as an enemy of everyone else—the price of freedom, which ruthlessly makes everyone a self-made man. This may explain to some extent the way in which the US faced the virus: ignorance going hand in hand with a combination of fear and self-defence. Concrete: a long time of ignoring the dangers; and a worrying increase in the sale of weapons: *'Handguns accounted for a huge jump in purchases. Estimated handgun sales increased 91.1% year-over-year, versus a 73.6% jump in long-gun sales, according to the SAAF data.*

As the coronavirus spread in March and more states ordered residents to stay at home, gun stores all over the country reported high sales volumes. Some even had to limit purchasing because they were running out of certain models"

(Druzin 1.4. 2020; 14/10/2023)

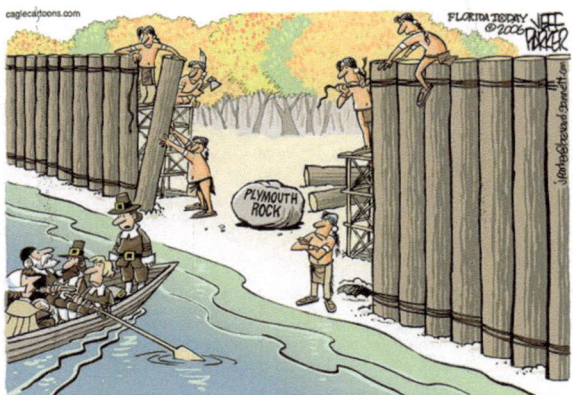

"THEY SAY THEY'RE BUILDING A WALL BECAUSE TOO MANY OF US ENTER ILLEGALLY AND WON'T LEARN THEIR LANGUAGE OR ASSIMILATE INTO THEIR CULTURE..."

Fig. 13.3 Migration, Assimilation and Power

Although arguments based on the notion of 'national character' have to be treated
with care—this being even more true if based on a small sample, without intro-
ducing any control variable as class, gender, religion .... Still, even this may
make at least thinking—finally the question of prejudice is a tricky one, as there
is some judice, i.e. some judication, some preceding judgement—a perpetuation
can hardly be avoided as the process of civilisation is one that is concerned
with the perpetuation of socialisation emerging from the conditions it creates in
the preceding stages of development—the irresolvable problem of the grandfa-
ther paradox that makes it so difficult to reach the other side where the grass
is always greener, not least as part of this civilising process is about social dis-
tancing. The problems of social science are not least consequence of a lack of
communication—on a superficial level we find plenty of chitchat, the exchange of
data, the bean-counting of everything and the speculative combination of a variety of data. Terms and concepts are taken for granted while any serious debate
is postponed—methodology chapters and papers are frequently chapters that deal
in actual fact with methods, analysis is too often looking at 'facts', however forgetting that positivism is characterised by a fundamental lack of understanding
and law is obsessed with rules forgetting the problematique that a decision may
be absolutely lawful, though it is in the light of fundamental, social and human
rights awful.

References

Used Literature

Adorno, Theodor W. et altera, 1950: The Authoritarian Personality; New York: Harper & Brothers

Agamben, Giorgio, 2020 a: A che punto siamo? L'epidemia come politica; Macerata: Quodlibet srl

Agamben, Giorgio, 2020 b: L'epidemia mostra che lo stato di eccezione è diventato la regola Intervista con Nicolas Truong, «Le Monde», 28 marzo 2020

Arendt, Hannah, 1958: Vita Activa oder Vom Tätigen Leben München/Zürich: Piper, 1967, Neuauflage: 1994

Becker, Ullrich et altera/Max Planck Institute for Social Policy and Social Law, November 2020: Protecting Livelihoods in the COVID-19 Crisis: Legal Comparison of Measures to Maintain Employment, the Economy and Social Protection. Updated Version; Munich: / Max Planck Institute for Social Policy and Social Law; working papers law, 7/2020

Becker, Ulrich, 2018: Soziales Entschädigungsrecht. Bestand, Grundsätze, Neuordnung; Baden-Baden: Nomos-Verlagsgesellschaft

Becker, Ulrich, November 2020 a: Social Policy and Social Law in Times of Crisis; in Becker, Ulrich et altera/Max Planck Institute for Social Policy and Social Law, November 2020: Protecting Livelihoods in the COVID-19 Crisis: Legal Comparison of Measures to Maintain Employment, the Economy and Social Protection. Updated Version; Munich: / Max Planck Institute for Social Policy and Social Law; working papers law, 7/2020: 9–21

Becker, Ulrich, November 2020 b: The Community Steps Up: Changing Responsibilities in Germany; in: Becker, Ullrich et altera/Max Planck Institute for Social Policy and Social Law, November 2020: Protecting Livelihoods in the COVID-19 Crisis: Legal Comparison of Measures to Maintain Employment, the Economy and Social Protection. Updated Version; Munich: /Max Planck Institute for Social Policy and Social Law; working papers law, 7/2020: 23–40

Berliner Senat, 2020: Pressemitteilung vom 14.12.2020; https://www.berlin.de/rbmskzl/akt uelles/pressemitteilungen/2020/pressemitteilung.1030169.php; 12/07/2021

Birch, Kean, 2017: A Research Agenda For Neoliberalism; Cheltenham/Northampton: Edward Elgar

© The Editor(s) (if applicable) and The Author(s), under exclusive license to Springer Fachmedien Wiesbaden GmbH, part of Springer Nature 2023
P. Herrmann, *Pandemics as Matter of a System Crisis,* Prekarisierung und soziale Entkopplung – transdisziplinäre Studien,
https://doi.org/10.1007/978-3-658-43450-2

Blasberg, Anita, 2022: Der Verlust. Warum nicht nur meiner Mutter das Vertrauen in unser Land abhandenkam; Hamburg: Rowohlt

Böckenförde, Ernst Wolfgang, 1973: Die verfassungstheoretische Unterscheidung von Staat und Gesellschaft als Bedingung der individuellen Freiheit; Opladen: Westdeutscher Verlag

Böckenförde, Ernst-Wolfgang, 1967: Die Entstehung des Staates als Vorgang der Säkularisation, in: Buve, Sergius (Hg.): Säkularisation und Utopie. Ebracher Studien, Ernst Forsthoff zum 65. Geburtstag, Stuttgart: Kohlhammer, 75–94

Böhme, Stefan et altera, 2020: Die Bedeutung der regionalen Wirtschaftsstruktur für die Arbeitsmarkteffekte der Corona-Pandemie - Eine erste Einschätzung. IAB-Forschungsbericht, 15/2020; Nürnberg: IAB; http://doku.iab.de/forschungsbericht/2020/fb1520.pdf; 12.07.21

Boldt, Klaus/Hirn, Wolfgang, 31.10.2003, 18.00 hrs: Sabines Welt in: manager magazin 11/2003; https://www.manager-magazin.de/unternehmen/sabines-welt-a-27ed852e-0002-0001-0000-000028945810; 20/03/2023

Bourdieu, Pierre, 2000: Les structures sociales de l'Économie, Paris, Éditions du Seuil

Braudel, Fernand, 1987: Grammaire des Civilisations; Paris: Flammarion, 1993

Brever, Joe, 2016: This is How Capitalism Works; https://artplusmarketing.com/this-is-how-capitalism-actually-works-b2907d1b4d78; 15/09/2019

Bruckmeier, Kerstin/ d'Andria, Diego/Konle-Seidl, Regina, 28.05.2021: Social protection of atypical workers during the Covid-19 crisis; https://www.iab-forum.de/en/social-protection-of-atypical-workers-during-the-covid-19-crisis/; 02/07/2021

CDU, 1947: Ahlener Programm der CDU der britischen Zone vom 3. Februar 1947; https://www.kas.de/it/einzeltitel/-/content/das-ahlener-programm-der-cdu-der-britischen-zone-vom-3.-februar-1947; 15.06.21

Cicero: De Legibus (book 1, 18 - https://www.perseus.tufts.edu/hopper/text?doc=Perseus%3Atext%3A2007.01.0030%3Abook%3D1%3Asection%3D18; 03/09/2023

Compton, Kristin, 2023: Big Pharma and Medical Device Manufacturers; Edited By Emily Miller; Last Modified: January 26, 2023; DrugWatch; https://www.drugwatch.com/manufacturers/; 04/03/2023

Dibelius, Alexander, 27.3.2020: Basis des Wohlstands erodiert. Ex-Chef von Goldman Sachs: 'Der Shutdown macht mir mehr Angst als der Virus'; in: focus; https://www.focus.de/finanzen/boerse/basis-des-wohlstands-erodiert-finanzprofi-warnt-vor-shutdown-die-groesste-globale-rezession-seit-100-jahren-droht_id_11806990.html; 28/02/2023

Die Bundesregierung, 29.6.2020: Konjunkturpaket: Die Mehrwertsteuer sinkt - wichtige Fragen und Antworten; https://www.bundesregierung.de/breg-de/themen/coronavirus/faq-mehrwertsteuersenkung-1764364; 11/07/2021

Dittrich, Monika, 2016: German Spelling Reform. Nearly a cultural war; Goethe Institute; https://www.goethe.de/en/spr/mag/20802137.html; 25.3.2020

Doku - Undercover als Paketsklave; 8.3.2012; https://youtu.be/AwgChC5ZGP0; Lieferdienste - Wer zahlt für unsere Bequemlichkeit? | Könnes kämpft | WDR; https://youtu.be/vnaKhi42CqU; 16.12.2020; accessed 27/06/2021

Druzin, Hesath, 1.4.2020: Gun Sales Skyrocket In March On Pandemic Fears; Boise State Public Radio; https://gunsandamerica.org/story/20/04/01/gun-sales-skyrocket-in-march-on-pandemic-fears/; 14/10/2023

Eder, Sebastian, updated 17.05.2020–11:00: COVID-19 – Arzt im Interview: „Es gibt eine sehr starke soziale Komponente bei dieser Krankheit'; in: FAZ 27/02/2023

Emmerich, Klaus, 2010: In guter Verfassung? Warum das Grundgesetz auf den Pruefstand gehört; Berlin: Verlag Das Neue Berlin

Eribon, Didier, 2013: Returning to Reims; Introduction by George Chauncey Translated by Michael Lucey; Los Angeles: Semiotext(e); originally published as Retour à Reims. © Librairie Artheme Fayard, 2009

European Council, 26th of March, 2020: Joint statement of the Members of the European Council, Brussels 26th of March, 2020; https://www.consilium.europa.eu/media/43076/26-vc-euco-statement-en.pdf

Fenrich, Katrin, 2015: Deutsch-griechischer Reparationsstreit: Zwei plus vier gleich null; in: Legal Tribune Online, 18.02.2015 , https://www.lto.de/persistent/a_id/14715/; accessed 27.03.2023

France, Anatole, 1894 : Le lys rouge

Fraser, Nancy, 2012: Can society be commodities all the way down? Polanyian reflections on capitalist crisis; FMSH-WP-2012–18; HAL archives-ouvertes.fr; <halshs-00725060>

Fraser, Nancy, 2013: A Triple Movement? Parsing the Politics of Crisis after Polanyi; in: new left review 81 may-june

Freeman, Alan, 2019: Sound policy, sound theory, sound facts: A breath of fresh air from China. Foreword; in: Cheng Enfu/Wang Guijin/Zhu Kui, 2005/2019: The Creation of Value by Living Labour. A Normative and Empirical Study, Vol. I; Translating Editor Alan Freeman Sun Yexia; Istanbul et altera: Canut International Publishers; Originally published (in Chinese) by Shanghai University of Finance and Economics Press, 2005: 1–12

Fricke, Thomas, et altera, 2023: The State of a shifting paradigm. New Thinking, New Actors — On the State of an Emerging Socio-Economic Paradigm Shift in Germany and Beyond; [Berlin]: Forum New Economy

Fuller, Lon L., 1949: The Case of the Speluncean Explorers, in: Harvard Law Review. The Harvard Law Review Association. 62 (4): 616–645. doi:https://doi.org/10.2307/1336025. JSTOR 1336025

Ganslmeier, Martin, ARD, Stand: 22.06.2021 17:39 Uhr: EU-Wiederaufbaufonds. Knapp 26 Milliarden Euro für Deutschland; https://www.tagesschau.de/inland/deutschland-wieder aufbaufonds-vonderleyen-merkel-101.html; 11.07.21

Gaschke, Susanne, Aktualisiert am 29. November 2013, 21:21 Uhr: Die Ich-AG und der ARD; Quelle: in: DIE ZEIT 13/2003; https://www.zeit.de/2003/13/S_Christiansen-2/komplettansicht; 20.03.23

Gramsci, Antonio, 1930: Quaderni del carcere, vol. I: quaderni 1.5; Edizione Critica del Istituto Gramsci a Cura di Valentino Gerratana; Torino: Giulio Einaudi, 1975

Hamilton Gary G./Zheng, Wang: Introduction to Fei Xiaotong's From the Soil-The Foundations; University of California Press, 1992

Harris, Chris, 2016: Why do governments in Italy change so often?; https://www.euronews.com/2016/12/13/why-do-italian-governments-change-so-often)

Herrmann, Peter, 1994: Die Organisation. Eine Analyse der modernen Gesellschaft); Rheinfelden/Berlin: Schäuble

Herrmann, Peter, 1994: The Organisation. An analysis of the Modern Society [German original title: Die Organisation. Eine Analyse der modernen Gesellschaft]; Rheinfelden/ Berlin: Schäuble Verlag

Herrmann, Peter, 2021: Privatisation breaching human rights 3; 2021 China Europe Seminar on Human Rights. Covid-19 Pandemic and guarantee of the Right to Life and Health; China Society for Human Rights Studies/Huan Rights Institute at SWUPI; https://youtu. be/yqEEVIUuTvw; 13/07/2021

Herrmann, Peter, December 2018: About You – Bei Strafe des Frageverbots, ob man überhaupt ist; in: Tarantel. Zeitschrift der Ökologische Plattform bei DER LINKEN

Herrmann, Peter, December 2019: International Seminar on International Human Rights Mechanisms from A Cross-Cultural Perspective; Changsha (https://youtu.be/pmcsc7 P-MYc; 04/10/2023)

Herrmann, Peter: Time to say Good-bye; https://rozenbergquarterly.com/time-to-say-good-bye/

Herzog, Roman,26.4.1997: Aufbruch in 21. Jahrhundert. Speech in the Hotel Adlon, Berlin; https://www.bundespraesident.de/SharedDocs/Reden/DE/Roman-Herzog/Reden/ 1997/04/19970426_Rede.html; 19.03.23

HIST 234: Epidemics in Western Society Since 1600: https://oyc.yale.edu/history/hist-234/ lecture-1; 05/07/2023

IAB-Forum, 16.4.2020: European labour market dynamics after the outbreak of the Covid-19 crisis; Series 'COVID-19 crisis. Consequences for the Labour Market; https://www. iab-forum.de/en/european-labour-market-dynamics-after-the-outbreak-of-the-covid-19-crisis/; 12/07/21

IAB-Forum, 26.02.2021: Magazine of the Institute for Employment Research: The impact of the Covid-19 pandemic: evidence from a new establishment survey; Series 'COVID-19 Crisis: Consequences for the Labour Market'; https://www.iab-forum.de/en/the-impact-of-the-covid-19-pandemic-evidence-from-a-new-establishment-survey/; 12/07/2021

ILO, 2020: Global Wage Report 2020–21: Wages and minimum wages in the time of COVID-19; Geneva: ILO; https://www.ilo.org/wcmsp5/groups/public/---dgreports/---dcomm/---publ/documents/publication/wcms_762534.pdf; 15/07/2021

ILO: COVID 19 and the world of work; https://www.ilo.org/global/topics/coronavirus/lang--en/index.htm; 10/07/2021

ILO: COVID 19 and the world of work. Country Policy Responses; https://www.ilo.org/glo bal/topics/coronavirus/regional-country/country-responses/lang--en/index.htm#DE; 13/ 07/2021

Jorgensen, Paul D., 2013: Pharmaceuticals, Political Money, and Public Policy: A Theoretical and Empirical Agenda. Journal of Law, Medicine & Ethics, 41(3), 561-570. doi:https://doi.org/10.1111/jlme.12065

Kant, Immanuel, 1779: Über ein vermeintes Recht aus Menschenliebe zu lügen; Kant Akademie Ausgabe VIII: 426; https://korpora.zim.uni-duisburg-essen.de/Kant/aa08/425. html; 15.06.21

Kant, Immanuel, 1785: Grounding for the Metaphysics of Morals

Klenner, Hermann, 2009: Nachgedachtes, Vorgedachtes; in: Klartexte. Beitraege zur Geschichtsdebatte; eds. Ellen Brombacher et altera; Berlin: Verlag Das Neue Berlin: 11–15

Kofler, Leo, 1954/55: Marxistischer und stalinistischer Marxismus; in: Zur Kritik bürgerlicher Freiheit. Ausgewählte politisch-philosophische Texte eines marxistischen Einzelgängers; Hamburg: VSA-Verlag, 2000; 40–67

Kohl, Helmut, 1983: Erklärung der Bundesregierung; Deutscher Bundestag — 10. Wahlperiode — Stenographischer Bericht. 4. Sitzung. Bonn, Mittwoch, den 4. Mai 1983; https://dserver.bundestag.de/btp/10/10004.pdf; 19.03.23

Kohl, Helmut, 1990: Der entscheidende Schritt auf dem Weg in die gemeinsame Zukunft der Deutschen. Fernsehansprache des Bundeskanzlers zum Inkrafttreten der Währungsunion am 1. Juli 1990; Presse- und Informationsamt der Bundesregierung, Bulletin Nr. 86, 3.7.1990; https://www.chronik-der-mauer.de/material/180417/fernsehansprache-von-bundeskanzler-helmut-kohl-zum-inkrafttreten-der-waehrungsunion-1-juli-1990; 30/06/21

Kreilinger, Verena/Zeller, Christian, 21.3.2020: Corona-Pandemie — eine historische Wende Gesundheitswesen gesellschaftlich aneignen, Produktion kurzzeitig und geplant runterfahren! (gegenüber der Version vom 20. März leicht korrigiert und Abbildungen aktualisiert); http://www.oekosoz.org/2020/03/corona-pandemie-eine-historische-wende; 23.3.2020

Kurbjuweit, Dirk, 2010: Der „Wutbürger'. Stuttgart 21 und die Sarrazin-Debatte: Warum die Deutschen so viel protestieren; in: Der Spiegel 41/2010: 26 f.

Landsberg, Gerd, March 11th, 2020: Schließung von Krankenhäusern überdenken; Interview. SWR Aktuell; https://www.dstgb.de/themen/coronavirus/aktuelles/schliessung-von-krankenhaeusern-ueberdenken/; 11.07.21

Lederer, Klaus, 3.3.2021: Spiegel 'Spitzengespraech' mit Berlins Kultursenator Lederer; https://www.spiegel.de/politik/deutschland/klaus-lederer-die-linke-im-spiegel-spitzengespraech-der-albtraum-aller-vermieter-a-03f4e74a-80bd-45bc-bcdc-6d807cb939f7; 12/07/2021

Lessing, Gotthold Ephraim, 1769: Wie die Alten den Tod gebildet. Eine Untersuchung; in: Lessings Werke in sechs Baenden; Band 5; Berlin: Bibliographische Anstalt; without date: 183–226

Liessmann, Konrad Paul, 25.1.2021: Philosoph: Tun uns schwer, die Pandemie als Pandemie zu begreifen. Corona als persönliche Kränkung. Konrad Paul Liessmann im Gespräch mit Christiane Florin; https://www.deutschlandfunk.de/corona-als-persoenliche-kraenkung-philosoph-tun-uns-schwer.886.de.html?dram:article_id=491345; 30/06/2021

Luhmann, Niklas, 1993: Das Recht der Gesellschaft; Frankfurt/M.; First English edition: Law as Social System; Translated by Klaus A. Ziegert; Oxford: Oxford University Press, 2004

Machiavelli, Niccolò,1632: Il Principe; Torino: Einaudi 1961

Malik, Kenan, 2014: The Quest for a Moral Compass; Published by arrangement with Atlantic Books, Ltd; First Melville House printing; Brooklyn/London

Marcuse, Herbert, 1966: Der Mensch in einer sozialisierten Welt. Aufnahme: 03.10.1966, BR Technik: Schmitt Laufzeit: 47:13; CD 2: track 1: 2.45 min; from: Der Mensch in einer sozialisierten Welt. Originalvorträge von Herbert Marcuse. Autor: Herbert Marcuse. Sprecher: Herbert Marcuse. Aus der Reihe: O-Ton-Wissenschaft. Thema: Soziologie, Wissenschaft. 4 CDs - ca. 200 Minuten

Marshall, T.M., 1950: 'Citizenship and Social Class' in Citizenship and Social Class; T.H. Marshall/Tom Bottomore; London et altera: Pluto Press 1992

Marx, Karl, 1852: The Eighteenth Brumaire of Louis Bonaparte; in: Karl Marx Frederick Engels. Collected Works, Volume 11: Marx Engels 1851–53; Lawrence&Wishart:
Electric Books, 2012; 103–197

Marx, Karl, 1857–61: Economic Manuscripts Of 1857–1858. [First Version of Capital]; in:
Karl Marx Frederick Engels: Volume 28: Marx 1857–61; London: Lawrence & Wishart,
2010

Marx, Karl, 1867: Capital Volume One; in: Karl Marx. Frederick Engels. Collected Works,
volume 35; London: Lawrence&Wishart 1996

Marx, Karl, 1890: Das Kapital. Kritik der politischen Ökonomie. Erster Band. In: Marx-
Engels-Werke (MEW), Bd. 23. Berlin 1956 ff.

Marya, Rupa/Patel, Raj2021: Inflamed: Deep Medicine and the Anatomy of Injustice; Allen
Lane

McDonald, Aleecia M./Cranor, Lorrie Faith: 2008: The Cost of Reading Privacy Policies; https://kb.osu.edu/bitstream/handle/1811/72839/ISJLP_V4N3_543.pdf?sequence=
1&isAllowed=y; 08/01/19; S: A Journal of Law and Policy for the Information Society,
vol. 4, no. 3 (2008), 543–568.

McEwan, Ian, 2019; Machines Like Me and People Like You; New York: Anchor Books

Merkel, Angela, 11.03.2020: BUNDESPRESSEKONFERENZ; Angela Merkel, Jens Spahn,
Lothar Wieler – BPK zum Coronavirus; uncorrected transcript from https://youtu.be/kPG
T9pFIu8k; 05/07/21

Merkel, Angela, 2015: Statement by Angela Merkel during the press conference, 31.08.2015;
https://youtu.be/kDQki0MMFh4; 30/06/2021

Merkel, Angela, 24.3.2021: 27340 f Deutscher Bundestag – 19. Wahlperiode – 217. Sitzung.
Berlin, Mittwoch, den 24. März 2021; https://dserver.bundestag.de/btp/19/19217.pdf#P.
27340; https://dserver.bundestag.de/btp/19/19217.pdf#P.27341; 18/06/2021

Merkel, Angela, 28. 9. 2010: Rede auf dem BDI-Tag der Deutschen Industrie in Berlin; in:
Bulletin der Bundesregierung; 94–3; https://www.bundesregierung.de/resource/blob/975
954/771560/587d8ca69a6a72c74e91f54ec0c23331/94-3-bk-data.pdf?download=1;   20/
03/2023

Merkel, Angela, 28.3.2021: Anne Will - 28.03.2021 - Bundeskanzlerin Angela Merkel
(ARD); https://www.ndr.de/nachrichten/info/Angela-Merkel-zu-Gast-bei-Anne-Will,aud
io860140.html; 18/06/2021; https://youtu.be/UpEPnbgPkm0; youtube-transcript; mini-
mally edited; translated P.H.19/06/2021

Michels, Robert, 1915: Zur Soziologie des Parteiwesens in der modernen Demokratie:
Untersuchungen über die oligarchischen Tendenzen des Gruppenlebens; Leipzig, Verlag
Kröner, 1925

Milanovic, Branko, 2019: Capitalism Alone. The Future of the System that Rules the World;
Cambridge/London: The Belknap Press of Harvard University Press

Murray, Martin J., 1974: The Pharmaceutical Industry: A Study in Corporate Power; in:
International Journal of Health Services; 1974; 4(4): 625–640; doi:https://doi.org/10.
2190/M6YT-72J9-6LVV-FWG9

Nell-Breuning, Oswald, 1.3.1986: Subsidiaritaet in der Kirche; in: Stimmen der Zeit, Verlag
Herder; https://www.herder.de/stz/wiedergelesen/subsidiaritaet-in-der-kirche/; 10.07.21

O'Connor, James, 1973: The Fiscal Crisis of the State; New York: St. Martin's Press

OECD Berlin Centre and Institute for Employment Research – Research Institute of the Federal Employment Agency: 08/07/2021: 'Der Arbeitsmarkt nach Corona – was braucht

es für einen tragfähigen Aufschwung?; recording on youtube: https://youtu.be/XfRowJ 1avpM; 03/09/2023

Office re-entry is proving trickier than last year's abrupt exit; in: The Economist; 28/06/ 2021; https://www.economist.com/business/2021/06/28/office-re-entry-is-prov...cloud& utm_term=2021-06-28&utm_content=article-link-1&etear=nl_today_1; 29/06/2021

Paketfahrer - Ausgebeutet für den Online-Boom? I SWR betrifft; https://youtu.be/fF3WrY kELeo; Flüchtlinge als Paketzusteller - Deutsche Post am Limit - Doku 2018 (NEU in HD); 4.1.2018; https://youtu.be/xGCKNH4Tqk4; 27/06/2021

Pashukanis, Evgeny Bronislavovich, 1924: The General Theory of Law and Marxism in: Selected Writings on Marxism and Law; edited and with an Introduction by Piers Beirne/ Robert Sharlet; Translated by Peter B. Maggs; Foreword by John N. Hazard

Pashukanis, Evgeny Bronislavovich, 1924: The General Theory of Law and Marxism in: Selected Writings on Marxism and Law; edited and with an Introduction by Piers Beirne/ Robert Sharlet; Translated by Peter B. Maggs; Foreword by John N. Hazard; London et. altera: Academic Press, 1980

Pauly, Christoph/Dohmen, Frank, 2015: »Wer sind meine Freunde?« In: Der Spiegel 22/2015 [online]

Perke, Jan, 2021: Big Pharma & das Virus: Profite first: Das Beispiel Bayer; in: Bertz, D.F. (Ed.): Die Welt nach Corona. Von den Risiken des Kapitalismus, den Nebenwirkungen des Ausnahmezustands und der kommenden Gesellschaft; Berlin: Bertz + Fischer: 287–301

Pestalozzi, Heinrich, 1797: Meine Nachforschungen über den Gang der Natur in der Entwicklung des Menschengeschlechts; von dem Verfasser Lienhard und Gertrud; Zürich bei Heinrich Gessner, PSW 12, S. 1–221 (https://www.heinrich-pestalozzi.de/ werke/pestalozzi-volltexte-auf-dieser-website/1797-meine-nachforschungen/meine-nac hforschungen-37; 14.10.23)

Petersen, Thomas, IdA, updated 16.06.2021–05:53: Eine Mehrheit fühlt sich gegängelt; Allensbach Umfrage; in: FAZ; https://www.faz.net/aktuell/politik/inland/allensbach-umf rage-viele-zweifeln-an-meinungsfreiheit-in-deutschland-17390954.html;13/07/2021

Pistor, Katharina, 2019: The Code of Capital: How the Law Creates Wealth and Inequality (10th edn), Princeton University Press: X

Plitz, Christopher, 20.6.2021: Warum Einsamkeit krank macht – und was dagegen hilft in: Der Spiegel, 25/2021; https://www.spiegel.de/panorama/gesellschaft/isolation-wae hrend-corona-warum-einsamkeit-krank-macht-und-was-dagegen-hilft-a-ab2e1f23-0002-0001-0000-000177967157?context=issue; 27/06/2021

Polanyi, Karl, 1944: The Great Transformation: The Political and Economic Origins of Our Time; Boston: Beacon Press, 1957

Pollock, James, K, General Clay's Advisor on German Government, to the Chicago Council on Foreign Relations, June 9, 1947, quoted in: Woods Eisenberg, Carolyn, 1996: Drawing the line. The American decision to divide Germany, 1944–1949 Cambridge et altera: Cambridge University Press

Pope Leo XIII, 1891: Rerum Novarum Lettera Enciclica; https://www.vatican.va/con tent/leo-xiii/it/encyclicals/documents/hf_l-xiii_enc_15051891_rerum-novarum.html; 15/ 06/2021

Pope Pius XI, 1931: Lettera Enciclica Quadragesimo Anno Del Sommo Pontefice Pio Xi Ai Venerabili Fratelli Patriarchi, Primati, Arcivescovi, Vescovi E Agli Altri Ordinari Locali

Che Hanno Pace E Comunione Con La Sede Apostolica, Sulla Ricostruzione Dell'ordine Sociale Nel 40° Anniversario Della Rerum Novarum; https://www.vatican.va/content/pius-xi/it/encyclicals/documents/hf_p-xi_enc_19310515_quadragesimo-anno.html; 15/06/2021

praktischArzt » Medizinische Berufe » Krankenschwester Gehalt: was verdient eine Krankenschwester?; https://www.praktischarzt.de/medizinische-berufe/krankenschwester-gehalt/; 12/07/2021

Quadbeck, Eva, 29.12.2020, 12:55: Krankenhäusern helfen – Medizinisches Personal muss Gehalt bekommen; Redaktionsnetzwerk Deutschland; https://www.rnd.de/politik/krankenhausern-helfen-gehalter-zahlen-MNYD2TRSABCOVKD7SOI3RDO5EE.html; 12/07/2021

Rawls, John, 2001: Justice as Fairness: A Restatement, Cambridge, Massachusetts: Belknap Press

Reckwitz, Andreas, 2020: The Society of Singularities. Translated by Valentine A. Pakis; Cambridge: Polity; Original: 2017: Die Gesellschaft der Singularitäten; Berlin: Suhrkamp Verlag

Ridder, Helmut, 1951: Enteignung und Sozialisierung; in: Ungeschriebenes Verfassungsrecht. Enteignung und Sozialisierung. Verhandlungen der Tagung der Deutschen Staatsrechtslehrer zu Göttingen am 18. und 19. Oktober 1951. Mit einem Auszug aus der Aussprache. With contributions by: Ernst von Hippel, Alfred Voigt, Hans P. Ipsen and Helmut K. Ridder Volume 10 in the series Veröffentlichungen der Vereinigung der Deutschen Staatsrechtslehrer; 124–147; https://doi.org/10.1515/9783110900750; 22.09.21

Rudnicka, J./statista, 11.06.2021: Anzahl der Insolvenzverfahren insgesamt in Deutschland von März 2020 bis März 2021; https://de.statista.com/statistik/daten/studie/37122/umfrage/anzahl-der-insolvenzen-in-deutschland-insgesamt/#professional; 06/07/2021

Sablowski, Thomas, 2020: Klassenkämpfe in der Corona-Krise. Die Auseinandersetzung um die wirtschaftspolitischen Maßnahmen der Bundesregierung; in: PROKLA 200|50. Jahrgang . Nr 3 September 2020: 519–542; https://doi.org/10.32387/prokla.v50i200.1904

Scarpetta, Stefano/Carcillo, Stéphane, 08.07.2021: OECD Employment Outlook 2022. Navigating the COVID-19 crisis and recovery .OECD, IAB webinar; slides made available by the OECD

Schirrmacher, Frank, 2011: Buergerliche Werte. Ich beginne zu glauben, dass die Linke recht hat; in: FAZ; https://www.faz.net/aktuell/feuilleton/buergerliche-werte-ich-beginne-zu-glauben-dass-die-linke-recht-hat-11106162.html?printPagedArticle=true#pageIndex_2; 26/03/2023; Permalink: https://www.faz.net/-gqz-6m1ki

Schmid, Carlo, 1981: Erinnerungen; Wilhelm Goldmann Verlag

Schweizer Radio und Fernsehen; Swiss Radio and TV Broadcasting https://www.srf.ch/play/tv/sendung/sternstunde-philosophie?id=b7705a5d-4b68-4cb1-9404-03932cd8d569; 27/06/2021

Smith, Adam, 1776: An Inquiry into the Nature and Causes of the Wealth of Nations; Volume 1; Edited by R. H. Campbell and A. S. Skinner; textual editor W. B. Todd (The Glasgow Edition Of The Works And Correspondence Of Adam Smith, II); Indianapolis: Liberty Classics

Solty, Ingar, 1.3.2023: Linker Bellizismus. Knoten im Kopf. Die Aporien der linken und linksradikalen Befürworter von Waffenlieferungen in die Ukraine; Junge Welt, 51/

1.3.2023; https://www.jungewelt.de/artikel/445935.linker-bellizismus-knoten-im-kopf.
html?sstr=solty; 02/03/2023

Spinnen, Burkhard, 22.06.2007: Priesterin eines traurigen Rituals. Meinung; https://www.
welt.de/debatte/kommentare/article6069238/Priesterin-eines-traurigen-Rituals.html;
20.03.23

Stam, Claire, without date: Common Good; https://www.euractiv.com/section/coronavirus/
news/the-brief-common-good/; 12/03/20

Stimmenfang #163: Das Jahrzehnt der Wutbürger - von Stuttgart 21 bis Corona; https://www.
youtube.com/watch?v=ecSruHF7ETk; 15/07/2021

Streeck, Wolfgang July 2013: The Politics of Public Debt: Neoliberalism, Capitalist Devel-
opment, and the Restructuring of the State; MPIfG Discussion Paper 13/7; Max-Planck-
Institut für Gesellschaftsforschung, Köln/Max Planck Institute for the Study of Societies,
Cologne)

Tansey, Rachel, 9/2020: Power and Profit During a Pandemic. Why the Pharmaceutical
Industry Needs More Scrutiny Not Less; Corporate Europe Observatory; https://corpor
ateeurope.org/en/2020/09/power-and-profit-during-pandemic; 04/03/2023;

TV Doku: Schuften bis zum Umfallen - DHL Zusteller unter Druck – ZDFZoom;
24.10.2018; https://youtu.be/XMT54J2LpOA; 27/06/2021

Union pour l'Unité, 25/05/2021 : Politique des bâtiments de la Commission à Bruxelles.
Communiqué de presse; https://u4unity.eu/document3/communik_20210525.pdf; 01/07/
21

v.d. Leyen, Ursula, 12.3.2020: in: Corona-Hilfsprogramm der EU: Mühsam berechnete Milliarden - news.ORF.at; ORF; https://orf.at/stories/3157397/; 14/10/2023

van der Maesen, Laurent J. G.; Walker, Alan, 2012: Social Quality and Sustainability; in:
van der Maesen, Laurent J. G.; Walker, Alan (eds.): Social Quality. From Theory to
Indicators: Basingstoke: Palgrave Macmillan; 250–274

Varoufakis, Yanis, Feb 23, 2022: Our New Cloud-Based Ruling Class; in: Project Syndicate.
The World's Opinion Page; https://www.project-syndicate.org/commentary/new-ruling-
class-based-in-the-cloud-by-yanis-varoufakis-2022-02; 26/02/23

von Schirach, Ferdinand, 2017: Über die absolute Demokratie und das Recht (Festrede
in Salzburg, 2017); https://youtu.be/O08uAVDtWL4; 11.07.21; 12:39 – 17:43; slightly
edited/shortened

Abstract of the Federal Constitutional Court's Judgement of 15 January 1958 - 1 BvR 400/
51 [CODICES]; https://www.bundesverfassungsgericht.de/SharedDocs/Entscheidungen/
EN/1958/01/rs19580115_1bvr040051en.html;jsessionid=557A1A778F5E259217929
AFD688FDCBC.2_cid319; 20/03/2023

BGH, Urteil v. 14.7.2009, Az. VIII ZR 165/08

Bundesministerium für Finanzen Jahressteuergesetz 2020 (JStG 2020). 28.12.2020: Service;
https://www.bundesfinanzministerium.de/Content/DE/Gesetzestexte/Gesetze_Gesetze
svorhaben/Abteilungen/Abteilung_IV/19_Legislaturperiode/Gesetze_Verordnungen/
2020-12-28-JStG-2020/0-Gesetz.html; 01/07/21

BVerfG, 1977: [Public relations work of state organs at federal and Länder level] Judgement from the 02.03.1977 - 2 BvE 1/76; https://openjur.de/u/185031.html; 20.03.23;
translation P.H.)

BVerfG, Beschluss des Ersten Senats vom 15. Januar 1958 - 1 BvR 400/51 -, Rn. 1–75, http://
www.bverfg.de/e/rs19580115_1bvr040051.html

BVerfGE [Constitutional Court] – Luftsicherheitsgesetz; BVerfGE 30, 1 – Abhörurteil; BVerfGE abw. M. [dissenting opinion] 30, 173; BVerfGE 50, 166; BVerfGE 109, 133 – lebenslange Sicherheitsverwahrung

Chinese Constitution - http://www.npc.gov.cn/zgrdw/englishnpc/Constitution/2007-11/15/content_1372963.htm; 21/09/21

Constitution of South Africa - https://www.justice.gov.za/legislation/constitution/SAConstitution-web-eng.pdf; 21/09/21

Deutsche Rentenversicherung, 12.01.2021: Corona-Hilfe: Hinzuverdienstgrenze auch 2021 deutlich erhöht; https://www.deutsche-rentenversicherung.de/DRV/DE/Home/Corona_Blog/210112_hinzuverdienstgrenze_erhoeht.html;12/07/2021

Deutscher Bundestag 5. Wahlperiode Drucksache V/2291 Bundesrepublik Deutschland Der Bundeskanzler 1I/4 - 80402 - 6244/67 Bonn, den 16. November 1967∘ Entwurf eines Arbeitsförderungsgesetzes (AFG); https://dserver.bundestag.de/btd/05/022/0502291.pdf; 55)

Deutscher Bundestag Drucksache 19/18107 19. Wahlperiode 24.03.2020 Gesetzentwurf der Fraktionen der CDU/CSU und SPD Entwurf eines Gesetzes für den erleichterten Zugang zu sozialer Sicherung und zum Einsatz und zur Absicherung sozialer Dienstleister aufgrund des Coronavirus SARS-CoV-2 (Sozialschutz-Paket); https://dserver.bundestag.de/btd/19/181/1918107.pdf; 10.07.2021; bill in favour of easier access to social security and on the use and protection of social services providers due to the SARS-CoV-2 Coronavirus

Federal Constitutional Court, 2021: Risks of disadvantages for persons with disabilities in triage situations. Order of the First Senate of 16 December 2021 – 1 BvR 1541/20 -; http://www.bverfg.de/e/rs20211216_1bvr154120en.html; 04/03/2023

German basic law - http://www.npc.gov.cn/zgrdw/englishnpc/Constitution/2007-11/15/content_1372963.htm; 21/09/21

Gesetz zur Verhütung und Bekämpfung übertragbarer Krankheiten beim Menschen (Act on the Prevention and Control of Communicable Diseases in Humans) from 1961

Gesetzesbeschluss des Deutschen Bundestages Viertes Gesetz zum Schutz der Bevölkerung bei einer epidemischen Lage von nationaler Tragweite (Bundesrat Drucksache 315/21; 21.04.2021; https://www.bundesrat.de/SharedDocs/drucksachen/2021/0301-0400/315-21.pdf?__blob=publicationFile&v=1; 13/07/2021

https://www.bundesregierung.de/breg-en/search/all-day-care-at-primary-schools-to-be-exp anded-1911210; 13/07/2021; Gesetz zur Errichtung des Sondervermögens 'Ausbau ganztägiger Bildungs- und Betreuungsangebote für Kinder im Grundschulalter' (Ganztagsfinanzierungsgesetz - GaFG), BGBl, Nr. 61 vom 14. Dezember 2020; https://www.bgbl.de/xaver/bgbl/start.xav?startbk=Bundesanzeiger_BGBl&jumpTo=bgbl120s2865.pdf#__bgbl__%2F%2F*%5B%40attr_id%3D%27bgbl120s2865.pdf%27%5D__162625 8952260; 14/07/2021

Infektionsschutzgesetz – IfSG – Law on the Prevention and Control of Infectious Diseases in Humans (Protection against Infection Act – IfSG) (https://www.gesetze-im-internet.de/ifsg/index.html; 18/06/2021

Irish Constitution - http://www.irishstatutebook.ie/eli/cons/en#article43; 21/09/21

Joint statement of the Members of the European Council, Brussels 26th of March, 2020; https://www.consilium.europa.eu/media/43076/26-vc-euco-statement-en.pdf

LTO-Redaktion mit Material der dpa, 27.06.2023: Freiheitsstrafe auf Bewährung. Ex-Audi-Chef Stadler wegen Betrugs verurteilt; Urt. v. 27.06.2023, Az. W5 KLs 64 Js 22724/19; https://www.lto.de/recht/nachrichten/n/audi-diesel-manipulation-abgas-prozess-muenchen-rupert-stadler-urteil-bewaehrung/?utm_source=Eloqua&utm_content=WKDE_LEG_NSL_LTO_Daily_EM&utm_campaign=wkde_leg_mp_lto_daily_ab13.05.2019&utm_econtactid=CWOLT000034312644&utm_medium=email_newsletter&utm_crmid=; 29/06/2023

Notstandsgesetze ('Emergency Acts'), a term used for the 17th amendment of the Basic Law

Queen v Dudley and Stephens (1884) 14 QBD 273 DC (http://www.bailii.org/ew/cases/EWHC/QB/1884/2.html; 21/06/2021

Social Protection Package' (Deutscher Bundestag Drucksache 19/18107 19. Wahlperiode 24.03.2020 Gesetzentwurf der Fraktionen der CDU/CSU und SPD Entwurf eines Gesetzes für den erleichterten Zugang zu sozialer Sicherung und zum Einsatz und zur Absicherung sozialer Dienstleister aufgrund des Coronavirus SARS-CoV-2 (Sozialschutz-Paket); https://dserver.bundestag.de/btd/19/181/1918107.pdf; 10.07.2021 – bill in favour of easier access to social security and on the use and protection of social services providers due to the SARS-CoV-2 Coronavirus

Text, 1948: Text of Communique on the Six=Power London Conference on Western Germany; in: NYT, June 8, 1948, Page 14; https://www.nytimes.com/1948/06/08/archives/text-of-communique-on-the-sixpower-london-conference-on-western.html; 16/06/2021

Turkish constitution - https://global.tbmm.gov.tr/docs/constitution_en.pdf?TSPD_101_R0=08ffcef486ab2000df1865bd3b2f9ea48b8a6bfdcba4758e3ce02dbc1a48771cc4e74003d2eb949b080e49664e14300075b8d75e20265c9faf965f7e52e0892069ef7c3fd27bf7ed bacb1e3e338c680bb39a08931209243dacadf97a8ba3f60b; 21/09/21

domestic violence – https://www.msn.com/de-at/news/other/ausgangsbeschr-c3-a4nkungen-anstieg-der-gewalt-gegen-frauen-bef-c3-bcrchtet/ar-BB11121D; 28/03/2020

HIST 234 - HIST 234: Epidemics in Western Society Since 1600: https://oyc.yale.edu/history/hist-234/lecture-1; 05/07/2023

https://hemisphericinstitute.org/en/emisferica-14-1-expulsion/14-1-essays/the-border-s-crossed-us-too-the-intersections-of-native-american-and-immigrant-fights-for-justice-2.html#images-2; 05/07/2023

https://oyc.yale.edu/history/hist-234/lecture-12

https://www.abgeordnetenwatch.de/recherchen/informationsfreiheit/das-interne-strategiepapier-des-innenministeriums-zur-corona-pandemie; 02/03/2023

https://www.bbc.com/news/science-environment-57790040; 13/07/2021

https://www.bundesregierung.de/breg-de/themen/grundgesetz-fuer-die-bundesrepublik-deutschland-454028; 05.06.21

https://www.dw.com/de/willy-brandt-es-wächst-zusammen-was-zusammen-gehört/a-16431107; 02/09/2023

https://www.economist.com/graphic-detail/tracking-the-return-to-normalcy-after-covid-19; 13/07/2021

https://www.gesetze-im-internet.de/englisch_gg/englisch_gg.html; 21/09/21

https://www.msn.com/de-at/news/other/ausgangsbeschr-c3-a4nkungen-anstieg-der-gewalt-gegen-frauen-bef-c3-bcrchtet/ar-BB11121D; 28/03/2020

https://www.silber-salon.de/%C3%BCber; 27.06.21

Population China - https://www.worldometers.info/world-population/china-population/; 14/
    10/2023
https://www.silber-salon.de

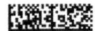